Person-Centred Healthcare Research

Person-Centred Healthcare Research

Edited by

Brendan McCormack
Queen Margaret University, Edinburgh, Scotland, UK

Sandra van Dulmen
NIVEL (Netherlands Institute for Health Services Research), Utrecht and Radboud University Medical Centre, Nijmegen, The Netherlands

Hilde Eide
University College of Southeast Norway, Drammen, Norway

Kirsti Skovdahl
University College of Southeast Norway, Drammen, Norway

Tom Eide
University College of Southeast Norway, Drammen, Norway

WILEY Blackwell

Registered Office(s)
John Wiley & Sons, Inc., 111 River Street, Hoboken, NJ 07030, USA
John Wiley & Sons Ltd, The Atrium, Southern Gate, Chichester, West Sussex, PO19 8SQ, UK

Editorial Office
The Atrium, Southern Gate, Chichester, West Sussex, PO19 8SQ, UK

For details of our global editorial offices, customer services, and more information about Wiley products visit us at www.wiley.com.

Library of Congress Cataloging-in-Publication Data

Names: McCormack, Brendan, editor. | Dulmen, A. M. van, editor. | Eide, Hilde, editor. |
    Skovdahl, Kirsti, 1964– editor. | Eide, Tom, editor.
Title: Person-centred healthcare research / edited by Brendan McCormack, Sandra van Dulmen,
    Hilde Eide, Kirsti Skovdahl, Tom Eide.
Description: Hoboken, NJ : Wiley, 2017. | Includes bibliographical references and index.
Identifiers: LCCN 2017026324 (print) | LCCN 2017026723 (ebook) | ISBN 9781119099611 (pdf) |
    ISBN 9781119099628 (epub) | ISBN 9781119099604 (pbk.)
Subjects: | MESH: Patient-Centered Care | Health Services Research
Classification: LCC R727.3 (ebook) | LCC R727.3 (print) | NLM W 84.7 | DDC 362.1–dc23
LC record available at https://lccn.loc.gov/2017026324

Cover image: © CYCV/Gettyimages
Cover design by Wiley

Set in 10/12pt Times by SPi Global, Pondicherry, India

Printed in the UK

Contents

Contributors

Rigmor C. Baraas PhD, BSc (Hons)
Professor
Faculty of Health and Social Sciences
University College of Southeast Norway
Drammen, Norway

Chyrell Bellamy PhD, MSW
Assistant Professor
Department of Psychiatry
Yale School of Medicine
New Haven, Connecticut, USA

Stian Biong DrPH, MPH, RN
Professor
Faculty of Health and Social Sciences
University College of Southeast Norway
Drammen, Norway

Marit Borg PhD
Professor
Faculty of Health and Social Sciences
University College of Southeast Norway
Drammen, Norway

Espen Brembo MA, RN
Assistant Professor/Lecturer
Department of Nursing and Health Sciences
University College of Southeast Norway
Drammen, Norway

Kristin Briseid MA (Political Science)
Assistant Professor
Faculty of Social Studies
VID Specialized University
Norway

Catherine Buckley PhD, MSc(Nursing),
BSc (Hons),
PGCert. Narrative Research, RGN
Practice Development Lecturer
Northridge House Education
and Research Centre, St Luke's Home
Cork, Ireland

Shaun Cardiff PhD, MSc, BEd, RGN
Senior Lecturer
School of People and Health Studies
Fontys University of Applied Sciences
The Netherlands

Larry Davidson PhD, MA(Psy), MA(Phil)
Professor of Psychology
School of Medicine and Institution for
Social and Policy Studies
Yale University
New Haven, Connecticut, USA

Jan Dewing PhD, MA, MN, BSc,
Dip Nurs Ed, Dip Nurs, RN
Sue Pembrey Chair in Nursing,
Director of The Centre for Person-Centred
Practice Research
Queen Margaret University
Edinburgh, Scotland, UK

Janne Dugstad MSc, BSc(Hons)
Director, The Science Centre
Health and Technology
Faculty of Health and Social Sciences
University College of Southeast Norway
Drammen, Norway

Sandra van Dulmen PhD
Programme Coordinator of
Communication in Healthcare
NIVEL (Netherlands Institute for Health
Services Research)
Utrecht, the Netherlands

Professor of Communication in Healthcare
Radboud University Medical Center
Nijmegen, the Netherlands

Professor II
Faculty of Health Sciences
University College of Southeast Norway
Drammen, Norway

Hilde Eide PhD, MA (Psy), RN
Professor in Communication and Health
Counselling, Research Director,
the Science Centre Health and Technology
Faculty of Health and Social Sciences
University College of Southeast Norway
Drammen, Norway

Tom Eide PhD
Professor of Leadership, Ethics and
Literature, and affiliated with the Science
Centre Health and Technology
Faculty of Health and Social Sciences
University College of Southeast Norway
Drammen, Norway

Lisbeth Fagerström PhD
Professor
Faculty of Health and Social Sciences
University College of Southeast Norway
Drammen, Norway

Åbo Akademi University
Vaasa, Finland

Elizabeth Flanagan PhD, MS
Research Scientist
Yale Program for Recovery and
Community Health
Yale University
New Haven, Connecticut, USA

Elisabeth Fosse PhD
Professor
Faculty of Health and Social Sciences
University College of Southeast Norway
Drammen, Norway

University of Bergen
Norway

Jon V. B. Gjelle MSc, BSc
PhD Candidate
Faculty of Health and Social Sciences
University College of Southeast Norway
Drammen, Norway

Kimberly Guy CNA
Peer Support Supervisor and Trainer
Yale Program for Recovery and
Community Health
Yale University
New Haven, Connecticut, USA

Linda Hafskjold MA (Clinical Health
Care), BSc (Radiography)
PhD Student
Faculty of Health and Social Sciences
University College of Southeast Norway
Drammen, Norway

Lene A. Hagen MPhil, BSc
PhD Candidate
Faculty of Health and Social Sciences
University College of Southeast Norway
Drammen, Norway

Gaby Jacobs PhD, MSc, PGCE, BSc
Professor in Person-Centred Practice
School of People and Health Studies
Fontys University of Applied Sciences
Eindhoven, the Netherlands

University for Humanistic Studies
Utrecht, the Netherlands

Famke van Lieshout PhD, MAsc, RN
Lecturer and Researcher
School of People and Health Studies
Fontys University of Applied Sciences
The Netherlands

Sylvia Määttä PhD, RN
Head, Department of Quality in
Healthcare
Western Region/Associate Professor
Institute of Health and Care Sciences
University of Gothenburg
Sweden

Brendan McCormack DPhil(Oxon),
RGN, RMN
Professor of Nursing/Head of The
Division of Nursing and Associate
Director
The Centre for Person-Centred
Practice Research
School of Health Sciences
Queen Margaret University
Edinburgh, Scotland, UK

Faculty of Health Sciences
University College of Southeast Norway
Drammen, Norway

Ottar Ness PhD
Professor
Faculty of Health and Social Sciences
University College of Southeast
Norway
Drammen, Norway

Maria O'Connell PhD, MA
Associate Professor of Psychiatry and
Director of Research and Evaluation
Yale Program for Recovery and
Community Health
Yale University
New Haven,
Connecticut, USA

Stina Öresland PhD, RNT
Associate Professor
Department of Nursing and Health
Sciences
University College of Southeast Norway
Drammen, Norway

Hilde R. Pedersen MSc, BSc
PhD Candidate
Faculty of Health and Social Sciences
University College of Southeast Norway
Drammen, Norway

Astrid Skatvedt PhD
Assistant Professor
Faculty of Social Science, Department of
Sociology and Social Work
University of Agder, Norway

Kirsti Skovdahl PhD, MA, BSC, RN
Professor, Programme Director of the PhD
Programme in Person-Centred
Healthcare
Faculty of Health and Social Sciences
University College of Southeast
Norway
Drammen, Norway

Ingun Stang PhD
Associate Professor
Department of Health,
Social and Welfare Studies
University College of Southeast Norway
Drammen, Norway

Vibeke Sundling PhD, MSc, BSc (Hons)
Associate Professor
Faculty of Health and Social Sciences
University College of Southeast Norway
Drammen, Norway

Angie Titchen DPhil(Oxon), MSc
(Rehabilitation Studies), Visiting Professor
Institute of Nursing and Health Research
Ulster University
Northern Ireland, UK

Steffen Torp PhD
Professor
Faculty of Health and Social Sciences
University College of Southeast Norway
Drammen, Norway

Caroline Williams MSc(Nursing),
PGDip(Facilitation), PGCE(FE),
BSc(Nurse Practitioner), RN
Professional and Practice Development Nurse
Hywel Dda University Health Board
Wales, UK

Teatske van der Zijpp PhD, MSc
Programme Lead, Technology in Care
School of People and Health Studies
Fontys University of Applied Sciences
The Netherlands

Introduction

Person-centred healthcare research is needed for service improvement and change. The world's first PhD programme in person-centred healthcare has run from autumn 2014 at the Faculty of Health Sciences at the University College of Southeast Norway (previously Buskerud University College). This was the start of a journey of international collaboration at our faculty, exploring different perspectives on what person-centred research presupposes and implies.

Patients and service users can feel vulnerable as they journey through the health system. Persons living with long-term health conditions, like mental health, substance abuse, dementia, stroke, chronic pain or diabetes have complex care needs that challenge health systems to respond in ways that keep the person at the centre of planning and decision-making. This challenge to person-centredness in healthcare is global. In Norway and beyond, the political vision is to create a health service that places the person, as the user of health services, in the centre of decision-making. The slogan is: 'No decision about me, without me'. In order to realise such a vision, our research needs to be interdisciplinary, informed by different perspectives and pluralistic regarding methodology, theory, and philosophy.

The Editors of this book reflect such a pluralistic approach to research. They are all leaders of and contributors to the PhD programme in person-centred healthcare at the University College of Southeast Norway. They are each passionate about research and whilst they each bring different methodological perspectives to their writing, what they share in common is a passion for 'the person' in health services research. The Editors, having brought together researchers from different fields and environments, encouraged new joint authorships, and together they have turned the writing of the book into an innovation process. Marvellous!

Person-centred healthcare research is a complex phenomenon. The book stimulates reflection and may serve as a guide for researchers at all levels. The PhD programme at the University College of Southeast Norway has a growing number of students studying person-centred healthcare from different perspectives using different methodologies. We are confident that this programme will have a significant influence on the advancement of new approaches to person-centred research and to our understanding of person-centredness itself – what I am sure is the beginning of a global community of person-centred doctoral researchers and post-doctoral researchers of the future. I am sure this book will be of great benefit to them and to all other researchers aiming at creating new knowledge to improve person-centredness in healthcare.

Dr Heidi Kapstad
Dean of the Faculty of Health and Social Sciences
University College of Southeast Norway

Foreword

International recognition is growing that person-centred healthcare offers a remedy to a continuing crisis in healthcare – a crisis in which clinicians and patients struggle to co-produce personalised and compassionate healthcare informed by, rather than based on, restricted scientific knowledge. Person-centred healthcare responds positively to this problem. It puts persons first in healthcare that bridges humanism and the sciences, including research. This book shows how health research on person-centred care can be person-centred. The Editors – world leaders in postgraduate education on person-centred healthcare – have unified international authors around the axial notion that research on person-centredness is fundamentally important, yet is insufficient unless it takes place in a person-centred manner.

Through conceptualising person-centredness and its foundations, the book first makes the case for conducting research to rehumanise modern healthcare in ways that balance the different warrants for healthcare decision-making. The book then suggests how to infuse this research – and, in turn, teaching, policy and practice – with assumptions, values and methodologies faithful to the philosophy of person-centredness. Examples of person-centred research are provided to bring to life this movement from research *on* person-centredness to such research *being* person-centred. Critical to the latter development is the guidance offered on using person-centred research designs and methodologies to deepen understanding and respect the personhood of research participants and researchers alike. Thus, the book helps to fill a gap within literature on health research methods and person-centredness. I enthusiastically commend this much-needed and highly original volume as an interdisciplinary resource for everyone producing or using person-centred research for health.

Associate Professor Stephen Buetow
Faculty of Medical and Health Sciences
University of Auckland
New Zealand
Associate-Editor, European Journal for Person-Centered Healthcare

Introduction to Section 1

PERSON-CENTREDNESS AND FOUNDATIONS OF PERSON-CENTRED RESEARCH

This section of the book is concerned with the philosophical and theoretical location of person-centred healthcare and person-centred research. It explores the importance of person-centred healthcare globally as well as the need for research that is undertaken through the philosophy of person-centredness. The case for person-centred research is made by drawing on a variety of theoretical and methodological perspectives, debating the relevance of existing methodologies and exploring research methods through a person-centred lens. Chapters in this section also illustrate examples of these theoretical and methodological perspectives and enable the reader to consider how these can be operationalised.

Person-Centred Healthcare Research, First Edition. Edited by Brendan McCormack, Sandra van Dulmen, Hilde Eide, Kirsti Skovdahl and Tom Eide.
© 2017 John Wiley & Sons Ltd. Published 2017 by John Wiley & Sons Ltd.

1 Person-Centredness in Healthcare Policy, Practice and Research

Brendan McCormack, Sandra van Dulmen, Hilde Eide, Kirsti Skovdahl and Tom Eide

INTRODUCTION

Twentieth century (western) societies are increasingly individualised. This is not only reflected in general politics, opinions and lifestyles but also in healthcare. Partly this is a result of an increased knowledge about the human genome, allowing for more individualised treatment plans ('personalised or precision medicine'), and partly because of scarce healthcare resources resulting in increased self-management and more patient responsibility for their own health. A welcome side effect of this individualisation is an increased attention to the person behind the patient and, related to this, more attention to individual needs and preferences in treatment and care. This person-centred movement is not new, but has so far been captured through discourses of patient-centredness (in contrast to doctor- or disease-centredness) and patients' rights, which already represent important paradigm shifts in healthcare. Person-centredness has, however, continued to develop and also incorporates concepts like positive health, well-being and individualised care planning as well as the inclusion of the person of the healthcare provider. Person-centredness can thus be summarised as promoting care of the person (of the totality of the person's health, including its ill and positive aspects), for the person (promoting the fulfilment of the person's life project), by the person (with clinicians extending themselves as full human beings with high ethical aspirations) and with the person (working respectfully, in collaboration and in an empowering manner) (Mezzich et al., 2009). Person-centredness implies recognition of the broad biological, social, psychological, cultural and spiritual dimensions of each person, their families and communities. The person-centred approach is closely linked to Carl Rogers' humanistic psychology and person-centred therapy (Rogers, 1961) with a focus on the fulfilment of personal potentials including sociability, the need to be with other human beings and a desire to know and be known by other people (the origins of person-centredness will be further explored in Chapter 2). It also includes being open to experience, being trusting and trustworthy, being curious about the world, being creative and compassionate. This perspective has been particularly influential in the field of dementia care.

Person-centredness has permeated all fields in healthcare. For example, person-centred nursing has been defined as an approach to practice that is established through the formation and fostering of healthful relationships between all care providers, patients/clients/families

Person-Centred Healthcare Research, First Edition. Edited by Brendan McCormack, Sandra van Dulmen, Hilde Eide, Kirsti Skovdahl and Tom Eide.

and significant others (McCormack and McCance, 2017). It is underpinned by values of respect for persons, individual right to self-determination, and mutual respect and understanding. Person-centred nursing practice is about developing, coordinating and providing healthcare services that respect the uniqueness of individuals by focusing on their beliefs, values, desires and wishes, independent of age, gender, social status, economy, faith, ethnicity and cultural background and in a context that includes collaborative and inclusive practices. In addition, person-centred nursing practice aims to plan and deliver care that takes account of the person's context including their social context, community networks, cultural norms and material supports. Person-centred medicine is anchored in a broad and holistic approach that is critical of the modern development of medicine, which has been dominated by reductionism, attention to disease, super-specialisation, commoditisation and commercialism (Mezzich *et al.*, 2009). These authors argue that this has resulted in less attention being paid to 'whole-person needs' and reduced focus on the ethical imperatives connected to promoting the autonomy, responsibility and dignity of every person involved.

Changes in the delivery of healthcare services have been significant over the past 25 years. The increasing demands on emergency services, reduction in the number of available hospital beds, shorter lengths of stay, increased throughput and the erosion of Health Services' commitment to the provision of continuing healthcare have all impacted on the way healthcare services are provided and the practice of healthcare professionals. In addition, the prevailing culture of consumerism has enabled a shift away from society's collective responsibility for the provision of an equitable and just healthcare system to one that is based on individual responsibility, increasingly more complex models of insurance-based services and a growth in healthcare as a private for-profit business.

The combined effects of these strategic changes to healthcare globally, major changes to the organisation of services, a dominant focus on standardisation and risk reduction with associated limits on the potential for creative practice have all had an impact on the ability of healthcare practitioners to develop person-centred approaches. McCormack (2001) suggested that there was a need for 'a cultural shift in philosophical values' in healthcare if authentic person-centred healthcare is to be realised for all persons. The following quote from one of the participants in McCormack's research highlighted the need for this shift:

> ...people need to be able to take on a different view of things and able to see a different kind of potential when the whole system is kind of set up in a particular way and how do you change it? Because you've got teachers and educators and you've got role models and supervisors and people in clinical settings who have all been socialised in this system and what I think it needs is actually a complete culture shift, a shift in philosophical values, to see people as people who have responsibility for their own health and come into a system that should not totally remove that, that kind of ownership...

Since then there have been significant developments globally in advancing person-centred healthcare within a dominant philosophy of people as persons who have responsibility for their own health.

PERSON-CENTREDNESS IN HEALTHCARE

The use of the term 'person-centred' has become increasingly common in health and social care services at a global level. While a cynical view would argue that the term is being used as a 'catch-all' for anything concerning high quality health and social care, an alternative perspective would suggest that it is representative of something more significant than this, i.e. a movement that has an explicit focus on humanising health services and ensuring that the person using health and social care services is at the centre of care delivery decision-making. This global focus on person-centredness has, as a consequence, resulted in a growing body of evidence supporting the processes and outcomes associated with person-centredness in health and social care.

Holding the person's values central in decision-making is essential to a person-centred approach to practice. Talking with patients and families about values and using the outcomes from these discussions as a means of evaluating how well their autonomy and self-determination is being respected is a useful vehicle for exploring the processes of care-giving as opposed to a focus on how well the care outcomes were achieved using, for instance, PROMS (Patient Reported Outcome Measures) and PREMS (Patient Reported Experience Measures). For example, the focus on achieving a short length of stay may not always be consistent with the values of the patient or family. In such situations, without the practitioner, patient and family clarifying their values base and its relationship to the goal of care, there is potential for conflict. The skill involved in balancing a duty of care to the patient while at the same time maintaining a focus on working with the 'best' evidence in care decisions is a significant challenge in person-centred healthcare. Maintaining the person's identity as central to care decisions and helping to maintain that in the sense of who they are in the context of their lives, i.e. their biography is a key pillar of person-centred practice (see Chapter 9 in this book for example). Rather than removing people from their biographies which has been the dominant ideology underpinning evidence-based practice (EBP), holding values as central allows a variety of possible 'futures' to emerge.

Of course, practising in this way poses challenges to healthcare practitioners who are largely educated and trained in a culture that emphasises professional control and expertise derived from autonomous decision-making. By controlling the outcome of care, healthcare practitioners are protected from needing to face the many difficulties and challenges associated with working with the patient's agenda – for example balancing the need for early discharge in order to maintain throughput, with the actual needs of the person. In addition, practitioners often lack the ability to appreciate the life skills that the person has because the patient is unable to demonstrate these skills in a hospital context, due to the attitudinal, organisational and socialisation constraints of healthcare organisations. Healthcare practitioners sometimes struggle to accept the choices that people might make, that is, if they had the choice to do so. Person-centred risk-taking is one of the biggest challenges that practitioners face in working in a person-centred way. The challenge in accepting person-centred risk assessment is that of balancing professional knowledge and personal knowledge, or, the blending of the professional with the personal. Healthcare practitioners need to be able to balance their technical competence and expertise and their professional caring roles with the patient's understanding of their own well-being and their potential future. This supports the central tenet of person-centredness being operationalised through an interconnected relationship between practitioner and patient.

Working in a person-centred way requires both personal bravery and supported development to make the necessary changes. Personal bravery arises from individual recognition of the need for change, often in organisational structures that do not support such openness or ongoing support of a learning culture. The healthcare educational system also needs to facilitate this development by including principles of person-centredness in education models, creating person-centred learning environments and developing collaborative practices between students and educators.

THE EVOLUTION OF PERSON-CENTREDNESS

There has been a proliferation of policy- and strategy-focused publications supporting the need for and development of person-centred cultures in healthcare. The Health Foundation has been instrumental in influencing many of these strategies and for ensuring that at least at the level of health systems, people are at the centre of care:

We want a more person-centred healthcare system, where people are supported to make informed decisions about and to successfully manage their own health and care, and choose when to invite others to act on their behalf ... We want healthcare services to understand and deliver care responsive to people's individual abilities, preferences, lifestyles and goals. (The Health Foundation, 2015a)

The Health Foundation has produced a range of resources to enable an increased understanding of person-centred care and to support its development in organisations (The Health Foundation, 2015b). However, despite its dominant focus on person-centredness, the focus continues to be on 'care' and less on how organisations create person-centred cultures.

The World Health Organization (WHO) has also promoted a person- and people-centred approach, with a global goal of humanising healthcare by ensuring that healthcare is rooted in universal principles of human rights and dignity, non-discrimination, participation and empowerment, access and equity, and a partnership of equals:

The overall vision for people-centred health care is one in which individuals, families and communities are served by and are able to participate in trusted health systems that respond to their needs in humane and holistic ways... (World Health Organization, 2007, p. 7)

Despite these notable advancements in the area of person-centredness there is much still to be done in developing health and social care cultures towards ones that truly place people at the centre of their care in order to achieve effective and meaningful outcomes. Richards, Coulter and Wicks (2015, p. 3) suggest that it is 'time to get real about delivering person-centred care' and argue that it requires a sea change in the mindset of health professionals and patients/clients alike. We would argue that a significant part of this sea change is the need to shift the discourse away from person-centred 'care' per se and to promote a unified discourse of person-centred 'cultures'. Person-centredness can only happen if there is a person-centred culture in place in care settings that enables staff to experience person-centredness and work and communicate in a person-centred way. With a focus on person-centred culture, we adopt the following definition of person-centredness:

... an approach to practice established through the formation and fostering of healthful relationships between all care providers, service users and others significant to them in their lives. It is underpinned by values of respect for persons, individual right to self-determination, mutual respect and understanding. It is enabled by cultures of empowerment that foster continuous approaches to practice development. (McCormack and McCance, 2017, p. 3)

Developing person-centred cultures in organisations requires a sustained commitment to practice development, service improvement and ways of working that embrace continuous feedback, reflection and engagement methods that enable all voices to be heard. This also has relevance for (person-centred) diagnosis and clinical care. However, it is still the case that this kind of culture change is slow to be achieved and there continues to be little evidence of wide-scale changes in health systems towards ways of working that privilege the person over organisational conformity. As Richards, Coulter and Wicks (2015, p. 3) argue, 'the challenge remains one of overcoming "system" inertia and paternalism'. However, even though wholescale shifts in systems may be slow, it is clear that person-centredness as a concept plays a significant role in shaping the thinking of policy makers and strategic planners in the way that health systems are evolving globally.

GLOBAL DEVELOPMENTS[1]

Reviewing person-centredness, person-centred practice and person-centred care developments around the world, it is fair to say that there has been an abundance of activity at the micro (e.g. practice initiatives and power shifts in the consulting room) and meso (e.g. support resources and education) levels of care delivery. We also note considerable developments at a macro level (e.g. national standards) most of which focus on informing strategic developments to inform the organisation of healthcare systems. However, it is also fair to say that there is a gap (or even a gulf!) between the strategic rhetoric of person-centredness and the realities of experience for patients, families, communities and staff.

Person-centredness as a concept has an intuitive 'fit' with the thinking of most healthcare practitioners, who despite everyday challenges have an overarching desire to 'do the right thing' for service users, families and communities. Being person-centred in a healthcare system that is dominated by business models of efficiency is a challenge for most practitioners. Holding the person at the centre of decision-making, when systems increasingly focus on productivity, places person-centredness in a precarious position in the minds of many practitioners. The mixed messages they receive about 'what matters', results in contradictions in determining priorities and ultimately an erosion of the quality of person-centredness experienced by service users. As a consequence, there has been a proliferation of developments and initiatives to improve the quality of care and make it more person-centred. Although there are 'pockets' of person-centred practice developments appearing in all fields of practice, there is still a tendency to view person-centred care as an approach that is most relevant to people living with dementia and those residing in residential care facilities. While there have been increasing developments in acute care, person-centredness here tends to be presented either fairly generically by teams of practitioners as core to shared values and beliefs or as part of a team philosophy, or as a technical approach to designing individualistic approaches to care planning and goal achievement. However, some significant examples of positive developments can be seen around the world and these need to be celebrated and encouraged.

In Australia, Perth Home Care Services (Western Australia) and Quality Healthcare (New South Wales) take a person-centred approach to providing homecare services for a range of clients such as those with disability or requiring dementia care, while in Tasmania a person-centred approach is used in delivering consistent palliative and end-of-life care (Tasmanian Department of Health and Human Services, 2014). The Essentials of Care is a state-wide nursing and midwifery programme in New South Wales (NSW) aimed at improving

---

[1] An elaborated version of this 'global developments' section can be found at:
  McCormack B *et al.* (2015) Person-centredness – the 'state' of the art. *International Practice Development Journal* http://www.fons.org/library/journal/volume5-person-centredness-suppl/article1

person-centred practice using a practice development approach (New South Wales Government Health, 2015) while Victoria Health has led the way in developing a guide and toolkit for implementing and evaluating person-centred approaches in caring for older people (Victoria State Government Department of Health and Human Services, 2012).

In Sweden, The University of Gothenburg Centre for Person-centred Care (GPCC) has developed a model based on three 'routines' in practice: Routine 1, initiating a partnership – patient narrative; Routine 2, working in partnership – shared decision-making; Routine 3, safeguarding the partnership – documenting the narrative (Ekman *et al.*, 2011). The approach has been applied in a range of settings with evidence of improved outcomes for patients and improved system efficiencies (Ekman *et al.*, 2011).

In The Netherlands, Vilans Dutch Expertise Centre for Long-Term Care has produced two Whitepapers on person-centred care in the last 2 years. The centre's goal is to help professionals improve care for people living with long-term conditions, vulnerable older people and people with disabilities, by providing practical guidelines and toolkits for person-centred care as well as offering advice and workshops/training programmes for staff. They focus on stimulating self-management, care plan development and models of shared decision-making. The Radboud University Medical Centre model for personalised care also places the patient central by customising care so that it fits the specific biological (including genetic), psychological and social make-up of the person. In the context of providing community nursing and supporting people to live independent lives in their own homes, the Dutch 'Buurtzorg model' of community nursing has achieved major international profiling. The model focuses on working in small teams of 6–12 nurses, working autonomously, working independently and having effective ICT support. Significant outcomes for patients, families and staff have been demonstrated (www.buurtzorgnederland.com). The model continues to grow and the underpinning principles are being adopted in many other countries.

The development of person-centredness in Norway lies in the series of challenges that are faced by health and welfare services, particularly the changes in population demographics and citizens with long-term health needs. Recommendations in several national policy documents in the mental health and substance abuse fields, in health promotion, rehabilitation, and innovation of healthcare services during the last decades have supported person-centredness. As in other western countries, the Norwegian health and social care services have been influenced by the global economic down-turn, being remodelled, redesigned and with an overall focus on primary care and public health. These reforms have been driven by the Norwegian Government Strategy – Coordination Reform (Norwegian Ministry of Health and Care Services, 2009). There are two central tracks for developing person-centredness and person-centred care in Norway; services for older people and services for persons with mental health and substance abuse problems. Within care for older people, the context has primarily been nursing homes and secondly community services. In nursing homes, nursing staff have increasingly integrated the principles and practices of person-centred care in collaboration with other professionals. There has also been a greater focus on person-centredness in the curriculum frameworks for nurses and other health professionals. Over the last decade, research around person-centredness and older people has increased, with the MEDCED-study (Testad *et al.*, 2015) at The Centre for Care Research, Western Region as an ongoing example. Advances in more person-centred mental health services have also emerged. In Norway, within mental health and substance abuse services, there is an increasing emphasis on person-centredness and person-centred practice. Human rights, recovery, empowerment and collaborative partnerships have been central areas of theoretical and practice development. The focus has been on user involvement, community support and tailored services. This new focus has influenced practice development, the curriculum frameworks for health and welfare professionals and the areas and contexts of research. In developing person-centredness and person-centred mental health and substance abuse care, three foci have emerged: (1) the perspective and involvement of service users; (2) recovery orientation of services; and (3) a multiprofessional and interdisciplinary context. In addition, The University College of Southeast Norway offers a PhD programme in Person-centred Healthcare, which is the first PhD programme of this kind in the world.

In the USA, most of the developments in person-centred care have been with older adults in long-term care but without dementia. This seems to be because of the focus on personal choice and preference and the difficulty of translating those values into the care of the person living with dementia. However, with the mandating of person-centred care in all Medicare and Medicaid funded nursing homes and the passing of the National Alzheimer's Plan Act (NAPA) in 2010 (Department of Health and Human Services, 2015) it is hoped that a more consistent change will be possible. Although with only limited resources allocated to care and advocacy in NAPA, there is greater emphasis on developing person-centredness for all older adults including those living with dementia. Unfortunately, there is a general belief amongst some providers that person-centred approaches are not good for the financial 'bottom line' with the concomitant impact on the adoption of person-centred practices. Several models of person-centred care have developed in the USA supported and coordinated by the Pioneer Network (2012), a cooperative network of state- or region-based coalitions of service providers. The Eden Alternative, Well-Spring, and the Green House models for communal long-term care facilities are probably the most well known and the ones that have conducted some evaluative research on outcomes for residents and staff. These models have focused a great deal on the importance of environment and in particular the arrangement of care in small groups, e.g. households within traditional nursing homes with Eden and Well-Spring, and purpose-built homes for small numbers of older adults. A promising research programme focused on person-centred communication in dementia care is developing models that aim to improve the overall quality of care (Williams *et al.*, 2016a,b,c).

At a macro level, person-centred thinking can be seen to influence a range of national developments and initiatives. Significant investment into strategic initiatives has been made in many countries around the world focusing on breaking down barriers that prevent people from accessing services, streamlining care delivery systems, nationalising evidence to underpin practices and make care safer. Key drivers in these strategic developments have been a universal commitment to ensuring the efficiency and effectiveness of services and minimising risk. For example, in South Australia a strategic state-wide approach has been undertaken with the release of *Caring with Kindness: The Nursing and Midwifery Professional Practice Framework* (South Australia Health, 2014) in September 2014. The framework aligns with the National Safety and Quality Health Service Standards (NSQHSS) (Australian Commission on Safety and Quality in Health Care, 2012), especially Standard 2 which highlights patients being placed at the centre of their own care and working in partnership. In Canada, The Alzheimer Society of Canada has initiated a 'culture change initiative' aimed at improving the experience of long-term care for people living with dementia and their families, and working with others to provide useful strategies, tools and tips that can help put the principles of person-centred care into practice (Alzheimer Society Canada, 2014). The work includes federally and provincially funded collaborative projects focused on education and training related to the principles and practices of person-centred care within home care and residential long-term care settings. In England the 'personalisation agenda' (Department of Health, 2010) in health and social care is a driving force for person-centred developments.

In Northern Ireland, within nursing and midwifery, there has been an explicit focus on person-centredness at a strategic level (Department of Health and Social Service and Public Safety, 2010). The theoretical development of a model for person-centred practice, which emerged from original research undertaken in Northern Ireland (McCormack and McCance, 2006, 2010, 2017), has influenced the discourse on developing person-centredness in practice. This has been further enhanced through a strategic shift in the country to an increased focus on improving the patient experience. One key initiative that has shaped this agenda was development of a set of standards aimed at improving the patient and client experience and a framework for measurement (Department of Health and Social Service and Public Safety, 2008). The focus on improving the patient experience is now recognised within the national commissioning directions as a priority for care delivery. This has provided increased impetus to embed a positive care experience at organisation and practice levels that reflects principles of person-centredness.

Person-centredness and person-centred care are at the heart of government health and social care policy in Scotland. *The Healthcare Quality Strategy for NHS Scotland* (Scottish Government, 2010) set out a clear vision and strategy for the development of a health service that is world leading and built on principles of care and compassion:

> *...What will make Scotland a world leader will be the combined effect of millions of individual care encounters that are consistently person-centred, clinically effective and safe, for every person, all the time... (Scottish Government, 2010, p. 1)*

This strategy set the direction for an ongoing programme of work that has focused on developing services that meet the needs of patients as persons and ensuring that care systems prioritise individual need. The *'Person-Centred Health and Care Collaborative'* has been a key platform of this activity managed through Healthcare Improvement Scotland (the government organisation responsible for healthcare improvement). This is a key part of a Scotland-wide programme of work aimed at improving health and care services so that they are focused on people, their families and carers. A variety of activities have happened through the Collaborative including learning events, online communities for discussion and debate, conferences and innovation 'cafés' as well as the development of a number of tools for person-centred care, such as the 'Five Must Do With Me Areas'. The Person-Centred Health and Care Collaborative has been a significant driving force behind many changes across the health system, including patient/client feedback systems, the development of quality standards, the education of all staff about person-centred approaches and of course influencing policy and everyday practices. In 2015, Scotland moved towards a fully integrated health and social care system and while this change is in itself a person-centred one, it also creates a range of new opportunities for extending the significance and reach of person-centred programmes of work.

In Malaysia, informed by the WHO policy framework for people-centred healthcare, services are being re-organised around people's need and expectations to make them more socially relevant and responsive, while producing better outcomes (World Health Organization, 2007). The Malaysian approach focuses on patients being empowered to and engaged in making decisions about their own healthcare with a particular focus on determining their own health outcomes. The Ministry of Health, Malaysia aims to 'help people to take individual responsibility and positive action for their health' and health providers are urged to enable people to participate in their own healthcare management, for example, by giving people treatment information and choices. The mission of the Ministry of Health, is to build a partnership for health, to facilitate and support people to attain fully their potential in health, motivate them to appreciate health as a valuable asset and take positive action to improve further and sustain their health status to enjoy a better quality of life. The translation of these strategies and policies into everyday practice is at a very early stage of development, but the potential of these developments to influence other countries of low to mid-range economic standing is significant.

The Institute of Health Improvement has been a significant player in promoting a strategic person-centred agenda and its focus on person- and family-centred care includes:

- developing care pathways that are co-designed and co-produced with individuals and their families;
- ensuring that people's care preferences are understood and honoured, including at the end of life;
- collaborating with partners on programmes designed to improve engagement, shared decision-making, and compassionate, empathic care; and
- working with partners to ensure that communities are supported to stay healthy and to provide care for their loved ones closer to home (http://www.ihi.org/Topics/PFCC/Pages/Overview.aspx).

However, evidence of sustainability of strategic initiatives to improve patient and family experiences continue to be lacking after 10 years of developments in this field. This lack of evidence of the sustainability of strategic developments highlights the challenges of translating person-centred policy and strategy into everyday practice. The extent to which the world of person-centredness has learned from other areas of work such as knowledge translation and implementation science is questionable, and it appears that in many cases the same mistakes continue to be made regarding 'how to get evidence into practice'. Some commentators have suggested that the service improvement and patient safety strategies have over-relied on 'data' to inform developments and neglected the importance and potential impact of relationships (cf. Martin, McKee and Dixon-Woods, 2015). Given the significance of relationships in person-centred theory this is indeed a significant 'oversight' and highlights the mismatch that sometimes exists between the conceptual and theoretical underpinnings of person-centredness and strategic developments in the field.

RESEARCH AND PERSON-CENTREDNESS

These global developments in person-centredness pose high demands on patients as well as healthcare providers. Research is needed to find the best and most effective ways to practise person-centredness. Research into person-centredness has increased significantly over the past 15 years. This is also noticeable in the launch of new scientific journals in this field, e.g. the *International Journal of Person Centered Medicine* (IJPCM) and the *European Journal for Person Centered Healthcare*. In these and other journals, published evidence has offered clarity to the meaning of the terms personhood and person-centredness (Dewing, 2004; Slater, 2006; Leplege *et al.*, 2007; Edvardsson, Fetherstonhaugh and Nay, 2010; McCormack and McCance, 2017) and offered insights into the cultural and contextual challenges associated with implementing a person-centred approach (McCormack *et al.*, 2008; McCormack and McCance, 2010; McMillan *et al.*, 2010; McCance *et al.*, 2013; Yalden *et al.*, 2013), the development of frameworks such as the Authentic Consciousness

Framework (McCormack, 2003), the Senses Framework (Nolan *et al.*, 2004), the Person-Centred Nursing Framework (McCormack and McCance, 2010), The Person-centred Practice Framework (McCormack and McCance, 2017) and Person-Centred Leadership Frameworks (Lynch, McCormack and McCance, 2011; Cardiff, 2016) alongside the application and testing of these frameworks in practice (Ryan *et al.*, 2008; McCance *et al.*, 2010; McCormack *et al.*, 2010a,b; McCormack, Dewing and McCance, 2011; Lynch, 2016). In addition, much more emphasis has been placed on outcome evaluation, including the development of tools to evaluate the relationships between person-centred processes and outcomes (Slater, McCormack and Bunting, 2009; McCormack *et al.*, 2010a; Smith *et al.*, 2010; Denford *et al.*, 2014; Slater, McCance and McCormack, 2015) and the relationship between person-centred care and particular health outcomes (van Dulmen, 2011; Ekman *et al.*, 2012; Olsson, 2014; Hansson *et al.*, 2015). There is, however, still much to be achieved in furthering outcome evaluation and this need was highlighted by the Health Foundation (de Silva, 2014) when the existence of 176 validated tools for evaluating person-centred care were reported, few of which were direct measures and all of which were proxies for person-centredness. Noteworthy too is the recently published state-of-the-art report from the Health Foundation, titled '*The State of Play in Person-Centred Care: A Pragmatic Review of How Person-Centred Care is Defined, Applied and Measured*' (Harding, Wait and Scrutton, 2016).

The examples of research that have an explicit focus on person-centredness reflect a growing movement in healthcare that has been generally referred to as 'the humanising of healthcare'. This is particularly significant in the world of medical practice, where the discourse of person-centred medicine is being given greater voice in the literature. Person-centred medicine places a particular focus on the centrality of the person and a challenge to the dominant Cartesian philosophy of reductionism and duality that has so heavily influenced medical teaching, research and practice throughout history – and as a consequence has influenced healthcare more generally. The focus on humanising medicine and healthcare is a challenge to such dualistic perspectives and instead places the significance of the person as a holistic being as the point of departure for decision-making, engagement and practice. Paying attention to the being of the person requires a more eclectic knowledge base by practitioners and an ability to contextualise knowledge in the life-world of the person. Shahar (2014) argues that while there is a growing focus on person-centredness and the centrality of the person, the reality is that many clinicians have lost the ability to connect with the personhood of persons and lose what they have learned about this in the transfer from the classroom to daily clinical care. While this is a particularly pessimistic perspective that Shahar offers, it is our contention that increasing numbers of doctors and other healthcare professionals are committed to a person-centred approach to their practice and are trying to find creative solutions to the challenges that Shahar poses. As we have already identified, there is a growing evidence base to guide us towards approaches to being person-centred in practice.

Person-centred practitioners do not focus on the resolution of individual and disconnected problems. Instead, they focus on the individual person's overall condition and coping resources through processes of 'negotiation' and 'informed flexibility' (McCormack and McCance, 2017). Focusing on their agendas rather than those of the practitioner or system facilitates person-centred decision-making (cf. Ekman *et al.*, 2011). This can be supported by eHealth and patient participatory designs (cf. van Bruinessen *et al.*, 2014). Engagement happens at a pace appropriate to the coping resources of individual patients and their perspectives on care practices. They further articulate an ability to engage at a level appropriate to the individual patient and are open to deal with the circumstances presented in the particular situations. They do not attempt to direct the agenda from their perspectives, but instead use patients' responses to determine next questions. Person-centred practitioners demonstrate the characteristic of being attuned to the particular situation that is shaped by patient responses without the overt reliance on conscious deliberation. They negotiate care plans and while they offer particular care inputs, these are usually negotiated with the patient. The patient's values are clearly recognised as important and 'mutuality' is demonstrated in the engagement between the practitioner and patient. Both participants articulate their values in the situation and there is evidence of patients respecting the practitioner's values as part of their decision-making process, suggesting that in those situations where patients' values are respected, they may be more receptive to advice and information from the practitioner (Ekman *et al.*, 2011). Other noteworthy examples include facilitating service users to be present in meetings of multidisciplinary teams and including service users in research applications and teams.

This perspective on the person-centred practitioner highlights the different approaches required in being person-centred compared with the standardised evidence-based medicine approach that has been reinforced as the key pillar of medical and healthcare decision-making. It represents a shift from 'one size fits all' based on standardised data to decision-making that starts with values, expectations, preferences, relationships, hopes and fears. It represents a rethinking about the meaning of 'professional expertise' where expertise focuses on the contextualisation of knowledge and evidence into the life world of the person. It represents a need for new skills in professional practice that facilitate meaningful engagement and coaching for health improvement rather than directing standardised interventions and ensuring compliance. In a recent editorial, Anjum *et al.* (2015, p. 427) posed a number of challenges to making these ways of practising a reality in healthcare practice:

- We lack adequate tools for handling the complexity of individuals, illness and evidence.
- We should avoid reduction to a single method, or at least we need more flexible methods.
- Specialists from different disciplines need to cooperate in order to best meet the complex needs of the patient.
- A correct understanding of biology includes the psychosocial. The biomedical model overlooks that biology is saturated with meaning.
- Phronesis, judgement and clinical experience must be given high epistemic value, since it is only in clinical situations that different types of evidence can be evaluated as a whole.
- Personal experience should be at the centre of a medical model.
- Theory is important in medicine. It is not sufficient to show how often an intervention works. We also need to understand how and why it works.
- The question of whether an intervention works occurs within a method, which might bring its own criteria of success. A challenge is to avoid relativism or 'anything goes'.

While some advances have been made in advancing these challenges, for example the replacement of the biomedical model with the biopsychosocial model of medicine (Engel, 1977), these challenges are very real as person-centred research moves forward and indeed many of them are picked up in this book. However, a further challenge we would suggest is that of advancing methodologies for person-centred research. Despite the global developments in person-centredness and the growth in research *into* person-centredness, little research has focused on research *as* person-centred. Doing research in a person-centred way continues to be under-represented in research reports and even the research into different aspects of person-centred healthcare usually fails to consider person-centred values in its underpinning methodology. There is little evidence of significant advancement in this regard and we believe that this is a key priority for research in person-centredness as we move the agenda forward.

A number of research centres have been established that demonstrate a commitment to advancing methodological expertise in person-centred research, such as the University of Buffalo Institute for Person Centred Care (http://www.buffalo.edu/ipcc/about-us/Partners. html), The Ulster University Person-centred Practice Research Centre (http://www.science. ulster.ac.uk/inhr/pcp/index.php), Queen Margaret University Edinburgh Centre for Person-centred Practice Research (http://www.qmu.ac.uk/research_knowledge/centre-for-person-centred-practice-research.aspx), Fontys University of Applied Sciences Knowledge Centre for Person-centred Evidence Based Practice (http://fontys.edu/home.htm) and the University of Gothenburg Centre for Person Centered Care (http://ckh.gu.se/english/research/centre-for-person-centered-care-gpcc). In addition, a new PhD programme in 'Person-Centred Health Care' is being provided by the Faculty of Health Sciences, at The University College of Southeast Norway. The aim of the programme is to support graduates who can carry out high-level research, professional development and evaluation of person-centred healthcare service provision within the area of health sciences, as well as advancing methodological developments in the field. In Europe, two organisations that work hard to implement person-centredness in policy, teaching and research are the European Society for Person Centered Healthcare (ESPCH) (http://www.pchealthcare.org.uk/) and the International College of Person-Centered Medicine (ICPCM) (http://www.personcenteredmedicine.org/).

SUMMARY AND BOOK STRUCTURE

Each of the chapters in this book pick up a number of the issues raised in this chapter. They highlight particular methodological developments, illustrate the challenges and successes associated with engaging in person-centred research and provide case examples of person-centred research in action. The book brings together work that we know is currently taking place in developing person-centred practice and advancing person-centred methodologies. We are very aware that this is an ever-changing field of research and there is much more work happening than can be included in a book like this – this is indeed something to be celebrated!

The book is divided into two sections.

Section 1: Person-Centredness and Foundations of Person-Centred Research is concerned with the philosophical and theoretical location of person-centred healthcare and person-centred research. It explores the importance of person-centred healthcare globally as well as the need for research that is undertaken through the philosophy of person-centredness. The case for person-centred research is made by drawing on a variety of theoretical perspectives, debating the relevance of existing methodologies and exploring research methods through a person-centred lens.

Section 2: Doing Person-Centred Research: Methods in Action will 'bring to life' the philosophical and theoretical perspectives discussed in Section 1. Researchers and academics who are engaged in person-centred research and who are every day, grappling with the challenges of doing research in a person-centred way, will lead the chapters.

REFERENCES

Alzheimer Society Canada (2014) *Culture Change towards Person-Centred Care.* Retrieved from: http://www.alzheimer.ca/en/We-can-help/Resources/For-health-care-professionals (accessed 1 February 2017).

Anjum, R.L., Copeland, S., Mumford, S. and Rocca, E. (2015) CauseHealth: integrating philosophical perspectives into person-centered healthcare. *European Journal for Person Centered Healthcare*, **3**, 427–430.

Australian Commission on Safety and Quality in Health Care (2012) *National Safety and Quality Health Service Standards.* Retrieved from: http://www.safetyandquality.gov.au/wp-content/uploads/2011/09/NSQHS-Standards-Sept-2012.pdf (accessed 1 February 2017).

van Bruinessen, I.R., van Weel-Baumgarten, E.M., Snippe, H.W. *et al.* (2014) Active patient participation in the development of an online intervention. *JMIR Research Protocols*, **3**, e59.

Cardiff, S. (2016) Person-centred nursing leadership, in *Person-Centred Practice in Nursing and Healthcare: Theory and Practice* (eds B. McCormack and T. McCance). John Wiley & Sons, Ltd, Chichester. pp. 86–98.

Denford, S., Frost, J., Dieppe, P. *et al.* (2014) Individualisation of drug treatments for patients with long-term conditions: a review of concepts. http://bmjopen.bmj.com/content/4/3/e004172.full.pdf+html (last accessed 1 February 2017).

Department of Health (2010) *Personalisation through Person-centred Planning.* Department of Health, London.

Department of Health and Human Services (2015) *National Plan to Address Alzheimer's Disease: 2015 Update.* Retrieved from: https://aspe.hhs.gov/national-plan-address-alzheimers-disease-2015-update (accessed 1 February 2017).

Department of Health and Social Service and Public Safety (2008) *Improving the Patient and Client Experience.* DHSSPS, Belfast.

Department of Health and Social Service and Public Safety (2010) *Partnership for Care 2010–2015.* DHSSPS, Belfast.

Dewing, J. (2004) Concerns relating to the application of frameworks to promote person-centredness in nursing with older people. *International Journal of Older People Nursing*, **13**, 39–44.

van Dulmen, S. (2011) The value of tailored communication for person-centred outcomes. *Journal of Evaluation in Clinical Practice*, **17**, 381–383.

Edvardsson, D., Fetherstonhaugh, D. and Nay, R. (2010) Promoting a continuation of self and normality: person-centred care as described by people with dementia, their family members and aged care staff. *Journal of Clinical Nursing*, **19**, 2611–2618.

Ekman, I., Swedberg, K., Taft, C. *et al.* (2011) Person-centered care — ready for prime time. *European Journal of Cardiovascular Nursing*, **10**, 248–251.

Ekman, I., Wolf, A., Olsson, L.E. *et al.* (2012) Effects of person-centred care in patients with chronic heart failure: the PCC-HF study. *European Heart Journal*, **33**, 1112–1129.

Engel, G.L. (1977) The need for a new medical model: a challenge for biomedicine. *Science*, **196**, 129–136.

Hansson, E., Ekman, I., Swedberg, K. *et al.* (2016) Person-centred care for patients with chronic heart failure – a cost-utility analysis. *European Journal of Cardiovascular Nursing*, **15**, 276–284.

Harding, E., Wait, S. and Scrutton, J. (2016) The state of play in person-centred care: a pragmatic review of how person-centred care is defined, applied and measured. http://www.healthpolicypartnership.com/example-work/person-centred-care/(accessed 1 February 2017).

Health Foundation (2015a) *Person-centred Care.* Retrieved from: http://www.health.org.uk/theme (accessed 1 February 2017).

Health Foundation (2015b) *Person-centred Care Resource Centre.* Retrieved from: http://personcentredcare.health.org.uk (accessed 1 February 2017).

Leplege, A., Gzil, F., Cammelli, M. *et al.* (2007) Person-centredness: conceptual and historical perspectives. *Disability and Rehabilitation*, **29**, 1555–1565.

Lynch, B., McCormack, B. and McCance, T. (2011) Development of a model of situational leadership in residential care for older people. *Journal of Nursing Management*, **19**, 1058–1069.

Lynch, B. (2015) Partnering for performance in situational leadership: a person-centred leadership approach. *International Practice Development Journal* **5** (Suppl) http://www.fons.org/Resources/Documents/Journal/Vol5Suppl/IPDJ_05(suppl)_05.pdf (accessed 1 February 2017).

McCance, T., Gribben, B., McCormack, B. and Laird, E. (2013) Promoting person-centred practice within acute care: the impact of culture and context on a facilitated practice development programme. *International Practice Development Journal*, **3**. http://www.fons.org/library/journal/volume3-issue1/article2 (accessed 1 February 2017).

McCance, T., Gribben, B., McCormack, B. and Mitchell, E. (2010) Improving the patient experience by exploring person-centred care in practice. Final Programme Report, Belfast Health and Social Care Trust, Belfast, Northern Ireland.

McCance, T. and Wilson, V. (2015) Using person-centred key performance indicators to improve paediatric services: an international venture. *International Practice Development Journal*, **5** (Special Issue on Person-centredness): Article 8. http://www.fons.org/library/journal/volume5-person-centredness-suppl/article8 (accessed 1 February 2017).

McCormack, B. (2001) *Negotiating Partnerships with Older People - A Person-Centred Approach*. Ashgate, Basingstoke.

McCormack, B. (2003) A conceptual framework for person-centred practice with older people. *International Journal of Nursing Practice*, **9**, 202–209.

McCormack, B., Dewing, J., Breslin, E. *et al.* (2010a) Developing person-centred practice: nursing outcomes arising from changes to the care environment in residential settings for older people. *International Journal of Older People Nursing*, **5**, 93–107.

McCormack, B., Dewing, J. and McCance, T. (2011) Developing person-centred care: addressing contextual challenges through practice development. *Online Journal of Issues in Nursing*, **16**, Manuscript 3. http://www.nursingworld.org/MainMenuCategories/ANAMarketplace/ANAPeriodicals/OJIN.aspx (accessed 1 February 2017).

McCormack, B., Karlsson, B., Dewing, J. and Lerdal, A. (2010b) Exploring person-centredness: a qualitative meta-synthesis of four studies. *Scandinavian Journal of Caring Sciences*, **24**, 620–634.

McCormack, B. and McCance, T. (2006) Development of a framework for person-centred nursing. *Journal of Advanced Nursing*, **56**, 1–8.

McCormack, B. and McCance, T. (2010) *Person-centred Nursing: Theory, Models and Methods*. Wiley Blackwell, Oxford.

McCormack, B. and McCance, T. (eds) (2017) *Person-centred Practice in Nursing and Healthcare: Theory and Practice*. Wiley Blackwell, Oxford.

McCormack, B., McCance, T., Slater, P. *et al.* (2008) Person-centred outcomes and cultural change, in *International Practice Development in Nursing and Healthcare* (eds K. Manley, B. McCormack and V. Wilson). Wiley Blackwell, Oxford. pp. 189–214.

McMillan, F., Kampers, D., Traynor, V. and Dewing, J. (2010) Person-centred caring as caring for country: an Indigenous Australian experience. *Dementia*, **9**, 1–5.

Martin, G., McKee, L. and Dixon-Woods, M. (2015) Beyond metrics? Utilizing 'soft intelligence' for healthcare quality and safety. *Social Science and Medicine*, **142**, 19–26.

Mezzich, J.E., Snaedal, J., van Weel, C. and Heath, I. (2009) The International Network for Person-centered Medicine: background and first steps. *World Medical Journal*, **55**, 104–107.

New South Wales Government Health (2015) *Essentials of Care*. Retrieved from: http://www.health.nsw.gov.au/nursing/projects/Pages/eoc.aspx (accessed 1 February 2017).

Nolan, M., Davies, S., Brown, J. *et al.* (2004) Beyond 'person-centred' care: a new vision for gerontological nursing. *International Journal of Older People Nursing*, **13**, 45–53.

Norwegian Ministry of Health and Care Services (2009) The Coordination Reform. Report No. 47 (2008–2009) to the Storting. Helse-og omsorgsdepartementet, Oslo.

Olsson, L.E., Karlsson, J., Berg, U. *et al.* (2014) Person-centred care compared with standardised care for patients undergoing total hip arthroplasty—a quasi-experimental study. *Journal of Orthopaedic Surgery and Research*, **9**, 95.

Pioneer Network (2012) *Request to Convey Information: Partnership to Improve Dementia Care in Nursing Homes*. Retrieved from: https://www.cms.gov/Medicare/Provider-Enrollment-and-Certification/SurveyCertificationGenInfo/Downloads/Survey-and-Cert-Letter-12-42-.pdf (accessed 1 February 2017).

Richards, T., Coulter, A. and Wicks, P. (2015) Time to deliver patient-centred care. *BMJ*, **350**, h530. Editorial. Retrieved from: http://www.bmj.com/content/350/bmj.h530 (accessed 1 February 2017).

Rogers, C. (1961). *On Becoming a Person*. Houghton Mifflin Co., Boston.

Ryan, T., Nolan, M., Reid, D. and Enderby, P. (2008) Using the Senses Framework to achieve relationship centred dementia care services. *Dementia*, **7**, 71–93.

Scottish Government (2010) *The Healthcare Quality Strategy for NHS Scotland.* Retrieved from: http://www.gov.scot/About/Performance/scotPerforms/objectives (accessed 1 February 2017).

Shahar, E. (2014) On medicine and science. *European Journal for Person Centered Healthcare,* **2,** 258–259.

de Silva, D. (2014) *Helping Measure Person-Centred Care: A Review of Evidence About Commonly Used Approaches and Tools Used to Help Measure Person-Centred Care.* The Health Foundation, London.

Slater, L. (2006) Person-centredness: a concept analysis. *Contemporary Nurse,* **23,** 135–144.

Slater, P., McCance, T. and McCormack, B. (2015) Exploring person-centred practice within acute hospital settings. *International Practice Development Journal.* http://www.fons.org/Resources/Documents/Journal/Vol5Suppl/IPDJ_05(suppl)_09.pdf (accessed 1 February 2017).

Slater, P., McCormack, B. and Bunting, B. (2009) The development and pilot testing of an instrument to measure nurses working environment: The Nursing Context Index. *Worldview of Evidence based Nursing,* **6,** 173–182.

Smith, S., Dewar, B., Pullin, S. and Tocher, R. (2010) Relationship centred outcomes focused on compassionate care for older people within in-patient care settings. *International Journal of Older People Nursing,* **5,** 128–136.

South Australia Health (2014) *Caring with Kindness: The Nursing and Midwifery Professional Practice Framework.* Retrieved from: http://www.sahealth.sa.gov.au/wps/wcm/connect/public+content/sa+health+internet/about+us/department+of+health/system+performance+division/nursing+and+midwifery+office/nursing+and+midwifery+professional+practice/caring+with+kindness+the+nursing+and+midwifery+professional+practice+framework (accessed 1 February 2017).

Tasmanian Government Department of Health and Human Services (2014) *An Approach to Healthy Dying in Tasmania: A Policy Framework.* Retrieved from: http://www.dhhs.tas.gov.au/__data/assets/pdf_file/0011/175169/DRAFT_for_comment_V_D_October_Healthy_Dying_Framework_Paper.pdf (accessed 1 February 2017).

Testad, I., Mekki, T., Førland, O. *et al.* (2016) Modeling and evaluating evidence-based continuing education program in nursing home dementia care (MEDCED)—training of care home staff to reduce use of restraint in care home residents with dementia. A cluster randomised controlled trial. *International Journal of Geriatric Psychiatry,* **31,** 24–32.

Victoria State Government Department of Health and Human Services (2012) *Best Care for Older People – The Toolkit.* Retrieved from: https://www2.health.vic.gov.au/hospitals-and-health-services/patient-care/older-people (accessed 1 February 2017).

Williams, K., Pennathur, P., Bossen, A. and Gloeckner, A. (2016a) Adapting telemonitoring technology use for older adults: a pilot study. *Research in Gerontological Nursing,* **9,** 17–23.

Williams, K.N., Perkhounkova, Y., Bossen, A. and Hein, M. (2016b) Nursing home staff intentions for learned communication skills: knowledge to practice. *Journal of Gerontological Nursing,* **42,** 26–34.

Williams, K.N., Perkhounkova, Y., Herman, R. and Bossen A. (2016c) A communication intervention to reduce resistiveness in dementia care: a cluster randomized controlled trial. *Gerontologist.* Apr 5. pii: gnw047.

World Health Organization (2007) *People-centred Health Care: A Policy Framework.* http://www.wpro.who.int/health_services/people_at_the_centre_of_care/documents/ENG-PCIPolicyFramework.pdf (accessed 1 February 2017).

Yalden, J., McCormack, B., O'Connor, M. and Hardy, S. (2013) Transforming end of life care using practice development: an arts-informed approach in residential aged care. *International Journal of Practice Development,* **3,** 1–18.

2 Philosophical Perspectives on Person-Centredness for Healthcare Research

Jan Dewing, Tom Eide and Brendan McCormack

INTRODUCTION

In order to theoretically contextualise research in person-centred healthcare, this chapter will provide an overview of the concept of person-centredness. It will draw on key philosophical ideas that have shaped our current thinking. A core principle underpinning this chapter is our commitment to developing clear philosophical foundations for person-centred research, although we are by no means advocating for any one 'single' position. We aim to show that coherent philosophical foundations are important for a number of reasons. Core to this, we subscribe to the view that having a thorough philosophical understanding of concepts and their relationships is essential to understanding the underpinning ontological and epistemological perspectives in different research paradigms. Having this knowledge enables the development of more rigorous research methodologies and ultimately the conduct of thoughtful and values-driven research in practice. Such research is more likely to develop new knowledge. We argue that there is a need for a more in-depth and perhaps multifaceted or even a complex understanding of the concept of person-centredness and of what person-centred practice research presupposes and implies.

The aims of this chapter are:

1. Explore core philosophical ideas of person and personhood.
2. Discuss the value and contribution of philosophical ideas in person-centred research.
3. Create opportunities for creative and critical thinking about research.

RESEARCH PARADIGMS

All research is based on assumptions about how we perceive the world and how we try to understand it. Although this can be achieved from many different perspectives, we never fully and completely know the world or even how best to understand it. Systematic thinking is the core business of philosophy, so it is philosophy that the researcher must turn to, to situate their research and to build connections with what is known and with what is yet to be

Person-Centred Healthcare Research, First Edition. Edited by Brendan McCormack, Sandra van Dulmen, Hilde Eide, Kirsti Skovdahl and Tom Eide.
© 2017 John Wiley & Sons Ltd. Published 2017 by John Wiley & Sons Ltd.

known. Our view of reality and 'being' is called ontology and the view of how we acquire knowledge is termed epistemology. Ontology is the starting point by which researchers start to imagine and construct a theoretical framework or paradigm for any significant research. At its core, ontology is the study of what we mean when we say something exists. Epistemology is the study of what we mean when we say we know something. For example, Crotty (1998, p. 3) defines epistemology as 'the theory of knowledge embedded in the theoretical perspective and thereby in the [research] methodology'. Together, ontological and epistemological assumptions make up a paradigm. The term paradigm, first termed by Kuhn (1972) refers to an overall theoretical research framework. An effective paradigm has elements of ontological and epistemological concepts as well as methodological principles that are sufficient and connected enough to each other to clearly situate the research. Further, the ontological assumptions or concepts should be seen to have informed the epistemological assumptions which in turn can be seen to inform the methodology. Together, they lead to a coherent research methods analysis and offer a framework for discussion of research findings. Table 2.1 shows an example of ontological and epistemological assumptions drawing on the critical paradigm and loosely drawing on ideas from Horkheimer, Habermas and Freire.

A framework derived from these principles, or something similar, would contain sufficient related concepts to develop a methodology and methods for research. For example, designing a research project to understand service-user experiences of an outpatient clinic for people surviving a stroke and drawing on the assumptions in Table 2.1, would consider the following methodological issues:

- What multiple realities need to be understood?
- Whose reality needs to be considered?
- Who are the key stakeholders in the research?
- What values will guide decision-making about data collection and analysis?
- How will data be presented in a way that respects the values of different stakeholders?
- How will the data be used to inform ongoing service developments?
- What will the role be of research participants?

These are some issues that need to be considered in designing a research methodology that is consistent with stated ontological and epistemological assumptions. However, these assumptions need to be further considered in the context of person-centred research. So, thinking about what person-centredness means is the obvious starting point in constructing a research paradigm for person-centred research.

Table 2.1   Ontological and epistemological assumptions from the critical paradigm.

Ontological assumptions	Epistemological assumptions
Social reality is defined by persons and is not fixed	Knowledge is socially constructed and there is no single truth
Social reality is influenced through media, institutions and society	Some forms of knowledge are valued more than others
Social activity is the outcome of persons' and groups' position in society and how much power they have	What counts as worthwhile knowledge is determined by the social and positional power of the 'creators' and 'owners' of knowledge
Advances in one person's or group's freedom and power usually leads to constraints in another's freedom and power	Knowledge is both a product and expression of power rather than truth

PERSON-CENTRED HEALTHCARE

Internationally, we can see that person-centredness is becoming more common in mainstream healthcare policies and in everyday healthcare talk. As McCormack and McCance (2017, p.1) point out person-centredness has had a long association with various philosophies, some applied sciences such as humanistic psychology and with professions such as nursing. There are many descriptions and definitions of person-centredness ranging from organisations such as the World Health Organization (2015) and the Health Foundation (2015) in the UK, to individual researchers and authors (see this overview for example by McCormack *et al.*, 2015). Person-centredness in healthcare seems to have become something that is taken for granted, even though evidence shows it is hard to realise in practice and is not as well developed as we might imagine or claim.

Indeed, more and more healthcare providers now claim that person-centred care and services is exactly what they provide. Some are even looking for the next new idea to follow person-centredness. On the other hand, evidence continues to show that far from humanising healthcare, people receiving healthcare continue to have mixed or poor experiences. Instead, they often feel that they are not listened to, that their essential concerns and needs are not taken into account, that decisions are made that lie outside best interests and are made without their involvement. In parallel, the same goes for many healthcare professionals. According to their experience, many more people regardless of role and place in the system feel that they are often not listened to, that their concerns for the quality of care are overlooked, and that decisions are made above their heads without sufficient consideration of consequences for people in need of healthcare and the professions delivering the care.

At the heart of practice there is, we argue, a number of essentials that need to be addressed if we are to engage in rigorous person-centred research:

- The need for clarity about what person-centredness is.
- Understanding of how person-centredness differs from patient-centredness and other related concepts.
- Engagement with philosophical ideas on what person-centredness is about and what it means for research.

Nevertheless, it can be argued, that anyone who considers themselves to be a person-centred researcher needs to examine what being a person means as part of their ontology. For us this is a lifetime commitment and never ends. As person-centred researchers we subscribe to the view that having a thorough philosophical understanding of an idea or concept is essential to understanding the underpinning ontological and epistemological perspectives of different research paradigms. Having this knowledge enables the development of more rigorous and coherent research methodologies and ultimately an authentic, thoughtful and values-driven research in and about practice.

WHAT IS A PERSON?

There are multiple philosophical perspectives that can help answer this question and there are in fact several questions around the nature of personhood that are of interest to us in person-centred practice research. Briefly, 'personhood' is the technical term used to describe the attributes persons have or hold – also note here, that persons not people is the plural for person. For most of us 'person' (a moral and legal entity) is often and incorrectly used synonymously with 'human being' (member of a biological species). Rorty (1992) explains that humans are biologically complicated because we are 'just the sort of organisms that interpret and modify agency through their conception of themselves'. For example, is a human being who is a foetus a person, is a child with severe learning disabilities a person, is a human being who is in a persistent vegetative state a person? Is an older adult with advanced Alzheimer's disease a person? Is a human being who has had some of their legal rights formally removed a person? There are many variations that we can question ourselves on what we think, value and believe. Further, to complicate matters more, there are those who argue that (other) species of animals are also entitled to be regarded as persons (Singer, 2009). In particular, some of the great apes such as gorillas who have quite sophisticated social psychologies, might be entitled to be considered as a person. What about whales and dolphins – are they also persons? Further afield, if non-human life was found on other planets would you/we consider these entities be considered as persons?

The concept of the person is believed to originate from the Greek *prosopon* and the Latin *persōna*, meaning 'mask' or 'false face'. In Ancient Greek and later Roman theatre the actors of tragedies, comedies and satyr plays wore masks, often of wood or clay. The *prosopon* or the *persōna* was the role, character or the personage in the drama. It may also be related to the Latin *personare*, meaning 'to sound through', probably referring to the mask as something spoken through and perhaps amplifying the sound of the voice. The root of both the Greek and the Latin concept is probably the Etruscan word *phersu*, meaning 'mask'. The etymological roots of the word person, including both mask and the voice within the mask reminds us of the indeterminacy or ambiguity of the modern concept of the person, often understood simplistically as being a unique human being, without much consideration of tensions between, for instance a person's social appearance, his or her existential experience of self and/or the person as perceived or recognised by others.

Most writers on person-centredness in healthcare – psychology, nursing or medicine – refer to Carl Rogers and his person-centred approach to psychotherapy (Rogers, 1961) as the starting point of the development of modern person-centred thinking. However, the roots of person-centredness go far beyond his work. Some trace the earliest roots of person-centred thinking to ancient civilisations, both Eastern, such as Chinese and Ayurvedic, and Western, particularly ancient Greek (Mezzich *et al.*, 2009). In the *Nicomachean Ethics* Aristotle argues in accordance with Socrates and Plato that moral virtues, like justice, courage and temperance, are complex rational, emotional and social skills (Aristotle, 1985; Kraut, 2013). According to Aristotle a person has a series of lower capacities common with animals, like capacity for nutrition, motion and perception. But the human person is a *rational* animal, with the capacities of morality, rationality, friendship and love. Thus, some philosophers argue that it is these higher order attributes that make the human animal different to others. These attributes give humans the capacity to live a good or virtuous life. A school of philosophy known as virtue ethics focuses on what living a good life means. The aim of life is to achieve well-being either through *Hedonia* (doing what leads to the greatest happiness and least unhappiness in the short term) or *Eudiamonia* (happiness or human flourishing in the longer term). In order to live well, we need a proper appreciation of the way in which such goods as justice, friendship and pleasure fit together. We must acquire, through practice, those deliberative, emotional, and social skills that enable us to put our general understanding of well-being into practice in ways that are suitable to each occasion. If we use reason well, we live well as human beings; or, to be more precise, using reason well over the course of a full life is what happiness consists of (Kraut, 2013, 5f). Of course, much Greek philosophy was written by men and meant to apply only to men who at that time were considered to be the society. However, for Aristotle, although the emotions are not represented seperately, they had even greater importance, particularly in the moral life, our capacity for which Aristotle regarded as largely a result of learning to feel the right emotions in the right circumstances (de Soussa, 2014).

Deliberations of personhood often start by asking *'what attributes must a human being possess to be a person?'* Many have been suggested such as cognition, and subsets including intelligence, rational decision-making plus the capacity for understanding and speaking language, the ability to make moral judgments, consciousness, free will, creativity, self-awareness and a soul. Some philosophical thinkers, Rousseau and Kant for example, hold that there is a normative aspect to personhood. Thus, personhood is not simply about describing how humans are but how they/we ought to be. And it has been long held that we 'ought' to be rational and autonomous beings. Frankfurt (1971), similarly argues that free will is the determinant attribute. He wrote that the criteria for being a person are designed to capture those attributes that are the subject of our most humane concern with ourselves and the source of what we regard as most important and most problematical in our lives. Deliberations have been complicated by those who believe in determinism and those who believe in free will. Hume (Ayer, 1954) is an example of a philosopher who argued that free will and determinism are compatible. Hume cleverly argued that people are free as long as they are doing what they want to do. Rorty helps by explaining that persons are required to unify the capacity for choice with the capacities for action. Because persons are primary agents of principle, their integrity requires freedom; because they are judged liable, their powers must be autonomous. But when this criterion for personhood is carried to its extreme, the scope of agency can be seen to have limits. Can we, for example, control the actions of our minds or our souls (if indeed we believe we have one)? Most philosophers agree that an orientation towards understanding what is right and wrong, good and bad, just and unjust is an essential aspect of personhood. Even here this can exclude some humans. Further, it is recognised that humans have the ability to form strong evaluations about our desires, beliefs and feelings and hold the potential to transform them in different ways. Frankfurt (1971) constructs a hierarchy of desires and volitions. A first order desire is wanting to do something. Mostly every creature has this type of desire. 'I want to eat'. A second order desire is the want to be different, or to have different first order desires. This self-evaluation, Frankfurt says, is a mostly human trait. A step up from this is a second order volition, that is, when someone wants a certain desire to be their will. Non-human animals, however, are said to act on first level desires.

> *Besides wanting and choosing and being moved to do this or that, [humans] may also want to have (or not to have) certain desires and motives. They are capable of wanting to be different, in their preferences and purposes, from what they are. Many animals appear to have the capacity for what I shall call 'first-order desires' or 'desires of the first order,' which are simply desires to do or not to do one thing or another. No animal other than man, however, appears to have the capacity for reflective self-evaluation that is manifested in the formation of second-order desires. (Frankfurt, 1971)*

Similarly, Smith (2003) suggests that human beings have a distinct set of capacities that distinguishes them significantly from other animals on the planet. Despite the vast differences in and between cultures and across time, no matter how differently people narrate their lives and histories, there remains an underlying structure of human personhood that helps to create order and similarities. Smith further argues that humans are animals who have an inescapable moral and spiritual dimension. They cannot avoid a fundamental moral orientation in life and this, says Smith, has profound consequences for how researchers must study human beings.

While there are those who argue that persons should always be regarded as having objective, absolute and intrinsic worth (McCormack and McCance, 2010, p. 9), whether or not they also happen to be valued by themselves and/or others, others propose alternative ideas. As soon as we have any differences between humans and persons we need to ask who is to determine who is a person and to what degree, or what attributes entitle a human being to be or remain a person; the person her- or himself, or another person relating to this person, for instance a healthcare worker? And who decides what attributes are associated with personhood? For example, this dilemma can clearly be seen in Kitwood's (1997, p. 8) somewhat limited definition of personhood:

> *a standing or status that is bestowed upon one human being, by others, in the context of relationships and social being. It implies recognition, respect and trust. Both the according of personhood, and the failure to do so, have consequences that are empirically testable.*

While arguing personhood is absolute, Kitwood also advocates that personhood is a social status awarded by another or others. Thus we need to examine carefully ideas by the same and different theorists and philosophers for consistency. Kitwood was influenced by ideas in the philosophy of dialogue by Martin Buber (Buber, 1923). In turn, Buber, like many others later on, also refers to the Danish existentialist Søren Kierkegaard as a source of inspiration, especially his work *Either/Or*, on the necessity of making choices in order to become a person (Kierkegaard, 1843/1992). Thus it is often possible to create a trail back in time and establish what ideas and preceding philosopher(s) have been influential in someone's thinking and theorising.

APPLYING CONCEPTS OF 'PERSON' IN PERSON-CENTRED RESEARCH

In the remainder of our chapter we will set out one possible set of ideas or concepts that a researcher might decide to use as a basis of person-centred research. In other words, this is a conceptual model for organising how we think about persons and personhood. This example is something we have created for the purpose of this chapter. We do this for two reasons; first there are so many philosophical concepts by so many different philosophers that researchers could try to grapple with in their exploration of personhood or in setting out their research paradigm. Secondly, we wanted to show that a conceptual model is essential for researchers and that it can be done.

Imagine that after reading through several philosophical texts the following core concepts have been identified by the researcher:

- A person is never merely a means to an end (Kant).
- I Thou (Buber).
- The other person as an ethical demand (Løgstrup).
- Finding the other person where he is (Kierkegaard).
- Strangeness of the Other (Levinas).
- Potential for becoming (Rogers).

These concepts were identified by a mix of 'intuition'. It felt like they would be meaningful, even if the reasoning for why this might be was not clear at the point of discovery; because the ideas felt closely aligned with the researcher's own world views including their values and beliefs about persons and by structured reflection on the research topic and questions. In these processes, we can see the interplay between different types of knowing and knowledge and between ontology and epistemology. The concepts are a little unusual in that they come from different schools of philosophy. Therefore, the researcher needs to explore in more depth their understanding of each concept and how they relate to each other. If the core concepts were different for example, let's say they were based on some central themes all within Merleau-Ponty's philosophy (1962) (perception, bodily movement, habit, ambiguity, and relations with others), then the philosophical framework for the research would be different to our first example in a number of ways, although the process of exploration would be similar.

Through reading, the researcher would come to appreciate that for Kant an imperative of being a person was his second formulation in which he stated:

> *[To] Act in such a way that you treat humanity [die Menschheit], whether in your own person or in the person of any other, never merely as a means to an end, but always at the same time as an end.*

As an Enlightenment moral philosopher, Kant's aim was to come up with a precise rational statement of the principles on which our ordinary moral judgements are based. The judgements in question are supposed to be those any 'normal' adult human with capacity would accept (Johnson, 2008). In his *Grounding for the Metaphysics of Morals* (1785) Kant argues that moral requirements are based on a standard or principle of rationality he called the 'Categorical Imperative'. Kantian duty ethics is demanding in a number of respects, and the formulation of this categorical imperative might be considered as a fundamental defence of the intrinsic worth and dignity of every human being. It is noteworthy that, according to the categorical imperative, personhood is about the humanity, *die Menschheit*, in every single person, oneself as well as others, including an intrinsic right to be treated as an end in itself, and never merely as a means to another end. The categorical imperative can be found as an integral part of most contemporary professional ethics, medical ethics and bioethics, and for person-centred healthcare and research.

Løgstrup was a Danish philosopher and theologian. His most influential work was *The Ethical Demand* (1956), where he takes a relational moral position. According to Løgstrup – like Buber, Rogers and Levinas – the basic human condition is that of the encounter, which in Løgstrup's view puts the responsibility on both persons. In Løgstrup's view, basic trust is fundamental to human life, 'a sovereign expression of life' (*suveræn livsytring*). In *The Ethical Demand* (*Den Etiske Fordring*), Løgstrup (1956) develops an account of an ultimate moral demand in our relations in life, emerging from trust, arguing that trust comes before social norms or moral principles:

> *Trust is not of our own making; it is given. Our life is so constituted that it cannot be lived except as one person lays him or herself open to another person and puts him or herself into that person's hands either by showing or claiming trust. By our very attitude to another we help to shape that person's world. By our attitude to the other person we help to determine the scope and hue of his or her world; we make it large or small, bright or drab, rich or dull, threatening or secure. We help to shape his or her world not by theories and views but by our very attitude towards him or her. Herein lies the unarticulated and one might say anonymous demand that we take care of the life which trust has placed in our hands. (Løgstrup, 1956, p. 18)*

The researcher finds out that because we are in a position to influence, to some degree, how well another person's life goes for them (even in minor ways), we find ourselves in a position of power over them. Indeed, Løgstrup argues that because power is involved in every human relationship, we are always in advance compelled to decide whether to use our power over the other for serving the other or for serving ourselves (p. 53). This resonates strongly with the second formulation in Kantian duty ethics. For Løgstrup (1956, p. 44) the demand built into our relations with others is that we may need to act one-sidedly for the other's sake, not our own.

> *Everything which an individual has opportunity to say and do in relation to the other person is to be done and said not for his own sake but for the sake of him or her whose life is in his hand.*

It is interesting to note that Løgstrup stresses that the ethical demand is not necessarily identical with the other person's wishes or expectations. It may, in fact, require going against the wishes of another person. To recognise the ethical demand one needs 'to make use of one's full capacity for altruism, insight, imagination and understanding of life'.

However, this demand ultimately turns out to be unfulfillable for Løgstrup in the sense that 'what is demanded is that the demand should not have been necessary'. In other words, in any given situation where the ethical demand becomes necessary, the person has already failed to live up to it (p. 146); the person should simply have acted spontaneously with selfless concern for the other. Equally, Løgstrup contends that the nature of life means it can only be experienced when a person lays him or herself open to another person and puts him or herself into that person's hands either by showing or claiming trust. This also means vulnerability is a prerequisite to trust.

Kierkegaard was one of the most important single influences on Buber's thought. Coming from two different traditions, Judaism and Christianity, their views of human existence as encounter were quite similar. Buber, it would be established by the researcher, is best known for his 1923 book, *Ich und Du (I and Thou)*, which distinguishes between 'I-Thou' and 'I-It' modes of existence. Buber's ideas emphasised the whole person and dialogic intersubjectivity. In his later writings he defines a human as a being who faces an 'other' and constructs a world of mutual confirmations from the dual acts of distancing and relating. Buber characterises I-Thou relations as dialogical and I-It relations as monological. Buber explains that I-It relations are not just a turning away from the other but also a turning back on oneself 'Through the Thou a man becomes I' (1923, p. 28). To perceive the other as an It is to take them as a classified and hence predictable and malleable object that exists only as a part of one's own experiences. In contrast, in an I-Thou relation both participants exist as polarities of relation, whose centre lies in between. We should be careful here not to dismiss the usefulness of I-It relations in some situations. In fact, Buber argues that each Thou must sometimes turn into an It in relations when they become fixed and mechanical. However, the researcher might be wary of criticisms that Buber's work is sometimes regarded more as a work of spiritual inspiration than of philosophy.

For Kierkegaard, being person-centred means that we work with what matters to other person(s) and that we have a respect for the others' values and beliefs. To achieve this argues Kierkegaard, one must first and foremost take care to find the other; where (s)he is and begin there. This is the secret in the entire art of helping. Anyone who cannot do this is themselves under a delusion if they think they are able to help someone else. Thus, in order truly to help someone else, 'I' must certainly first and foremost understand what (s)he understands. Further, Kierkegaard proposes that all true helping begins with a humbling. The helper must first humble themselves under the person(s) they want to help and thereby understand that to help is not to dominate but to serve, that to help is not to be the most dominating but the most patient, that to help is a willingness for the time being to put up with being in the wrong and not understanding what the other understands.

At the same time, the researcher has included a core idea by Levinas; the other as a stranger. This idea can be really useful particularly in a time characterised by increasing intolerance towards the other and the conflict that can occur where differences exist and diversity is not valued. There are many similarities with Buber's idea of I-Thou. Indeed, Levinas was influenced by Buber's philosophical ideas. However, there are some important distinctions in their ideas to the point they argue against each other. For example, unlike Buber, Levinas suggests that the other precedes the 'I' and is the basis of ethics. It is unclear who is the other that produces responsibility in the 'I' and enables the 'I' to become an active human being. However, Buber suggests we start from oneself, but not to aim at oneself; to comprehend oneself, but not to be preoccupied with oneself. The researcher would need to think through the differences carefully and see how, if at all, they can be harmonised.

Finally, the person-centred approach is in part, historically closely linked to Carl Rogers' humanistic psychology and person-centred therapy (Rogers, 1961). He mainly developed his thinking through his own experience with clients in therapy. Early in his career as a researcher at the University of Chicago he was philosophically interested in the status of the person in therapy and science. Rogers' article, 'Persons or Science?' (1955) is probably the first account ever of being (or becoming) a person-centred researcher. Referring to Buber's I-Thou relationship, he concludes that it is possible to make the perspective of science and person meet:

For science too, at its inception, is an 'I-Thou' relationship with the world of perceived objects, just as therapy at its deepest is an 'I-Thou' relationship with a person or persons. And only as a subjective person can I enter either of these relationships.

Rogers has useful ideas to contribute to person-centred research, although they are by no means a requirement. Rogers has a focus on the fulfilment of personal potentials including sociability, the need to be with other human beings and a desire to know and be known by other persons. This includes being open to experience, being trusting and trustworthy, being curious about the world, being creative and compassionate (British Association for the Person-centred Approach, 2014). Of interest to us is that he proposes 10 questions including 'How can I create a helping relationship' and 'Can I meet the other individual as a person who is in process of *becoming*, or will I be bound by his past or by my past?' In that respect he refers to what Martin Buber said on the importance of confirming the other (Rogers, 1961, p. 55).

Having established a clear set of philosophical ideas that are coherent and consistent with the researcher's own world view, the researcher can move on to identifying clear methodological principles for their research. Many of these methodological principles are articulated further in the remaining chapters in Section 1 of this book and in Section 2 the reader can see many of these principles being applied in completed and on-going research.

CONCLUSION

An aim of person-centred healthcare research should be to explore and support the capacity and capability of person-centredness in healthcare on micro, meso as well as macro levels, i.e. on the levels of the individual healthcare receivers and providers, the level of the service organisation and leadership, and the system level of healthcare institution and policies. Philosophy possesses an evaluative aspect and as a form of knowledge has both moral principles and power; it helps us achieve a deeper level of understanding in our discoveries since philosophy seeks to understand the essence of things, human reason, human action and its intended and unintended consequences. There is an increasing number of so called person-centred studies being published that are supposedly underpinned by person-centred concepts and theories, but which continue to use research methods that do not match such concepts and theories and thus reinforce a disconnect between the reality of person-centred practice and research methods used to evaluate it. We need to ensure person-centred research is rigorous and contributes to methodological and theoretical development as well as answering immediate research questions. Thus the priorities for future theoretical development and progressing methodological rigour in person-centred research must lie in advancing clearly articulated theoretical frameworks to guide the planning, conduct and evaluation of rigour in person-centred healthcare research.

REFERENCES

Aristotle (1985) *Nicomachean Ethics*. Hackett, Indianapolis.

Ayer, A.J. (1954) Freedom and necessity. *Philosophical Essays*, reprinted in Watson (ed.) 1982, Macmillan, London. pp. 15–23.

British Association for the Person-centred Approach (2014) What is a person-centred approach? http://www.bapca.org.uk/about/what-is-it.html (accessed 1 February 2017).

Buber, M. (1923/37) *I and Thou* (trans. by Ronald Gregor Smith). T. and T. Clark, Edinburgh.

Crotty, M. (1998) *The Foundations of Social Research*. Sage, London.

Frankfurt, H.G. (1971) Freedom of the will and the concept of a person. *The Journal of Philosophy*, **68**, 5–7.

Health Foundation (2015) *Person-centred Care*. Retrieved from: http://www.health.org.uk/theme (accessed 1 February 2017).

Johnson, R. (2008) Kant's Moral Philosophy, in *Stanford Encyclopedia of Philosophy* (ed. E.N. Zalta). https://plato.stanford.edu/entries/kant-moral/.

Kant, I. (1785/1993) *Grounding for the Metaphysics of Morals*. Hackett, Indianapolis.

Kierkegaard, S. (1843/1992) *Either/Or: A Fragment of Life* [*Enten-Eller*, translation and introduction by Alasdair Hannay]. Penguin, London.

Kitwood, T. (1997) *Dementia Reconsidered – The Person Comes First*. Open University Press, Buckingham.

Kraut, R. (2013) Aristotle's Ethics, in *Stanford Encyclopedia of Philosophy* (ed. E.N. Zalta). https://plato.stanford.edu/archives/spr2016/entries/aristotle-ethics/.

Kuhn, T. (1972) *The Structure of Scientific Revolutions*. The University of Chicago Press, Chicago.

Løgstrup, K.E. (1956/97) *The Ethical Demand* (translation of *Den etiske fordring*). University of Notre Dame Press, Notre Dame and London.

McCormack, B., Borg, M., Cardiff, S. *et al.* (2015) Person-centredness – the 'state' of the art. *International Practice Development Journal*, http://www.fons.org/library/journal/volume5-person-centredness-suppl/article1.

McCormack, B. and McCance, T. (2010) *Person-Centred Nursing: Theory and Practice*. Wiley Blackwell, Oxford.

McCormack, B. and McCance, T. (2017) *Person-Centred Practice in Nursing and Health Care: Theory and Practice*, 2nd edition. Wiley Blackwell, Oxford.

Merleau-Ponty, M. (1962) *Phenomenology of Perception*, trans. Smith. Routledge and Kegan Paul, London.

Mezzich, J., Snaedal, J., van Weel, C. and Heath, I. (2009) The International Network for Person-centered Medicine: background and first steps. *World Medical Journal*, **55**, 104–107.

Rogers, C.R. (1955) Persons or science? A philosophical question. *American Psychologist*, **10**, 267–278.

Rogers, C.R. (1961) *On Becoming a Person: A Therapist's View of Psychotherapy*. Houghton Mifflin, Boston.

Rorty, A.O. (1992) *The Identities of Persons*. University of California Press, Oakland.

Singer, P. (2009) *Animal Liberation: A New Ethics for our Treatment of Animals*. Harper Perennial Modern Classics, New York.

Smith, C. (2003) *Moral Believing Animals: Human Personhood and Culture*. Oxford University Press, Oxford.

de Sousa, R. (2014) Emotion, in *Stanford Encyclopedia of Philosophy* (ed. E.N. Zalta). http://plato.stanford.edu/entries/emotion/

World Health Organization (2015) *Placing People and Communities at the Centre of Health Services. WHO Global Strategy on Integrated People Centred Health Services 2016–2026. Executive Summary*. World Health Organization, Geneva.

3 The Knowing and Being of Person-Centred Research Practice Across Worldviews: An Epistemological and Ontological Framework

Angie Titchen, Shaun Cardiff and Stian Biong

INTRODUCTION

There are at least three areas of philosophical study that rigorous person-centred researchers draw upon to articulate the assumptions underpinning their research methodology, design and practice. First, there are assumptions underpinning the construct of person-centredness and these have been well defined in the work of McCormack and McCance (2010), key concepts being respect, self-determination, reciprocity and mutuality. The second area of study is epistemology – the philosophical theory of knowledge that 'seeks to define knowledge, distinguish its principal varieties, identify its sources, and establish its limits' (Bullock and Trombley, 2000, p. 279). Epistemology is concerned with knowing through cognitive representation (Titchen and Ajjawi, 2010). The third area is ontology, defined as the theory or study of what really exists (Bullock and Trombley, 2000) and it is concerned with the nature of reality and human being in the world (Guba, 1990) and what it means to be a person, either as researcher or participant in the research. Reality and being in the world are often embodied and embedded in shared meanings, behaviours and practices and although this embodiment is about knowing, it has no mental representation (Titchen and Ajjawi, 2010). Collectively, these assumptions form the bedrock of person-centred research and they will influence every other assumption in the work from what determines reality to the view of the person and the world. Thus the bedrock shapes the outcome and the products of the research and imbues everything researchers do, not only in designing the study, but also in carrying it out. This includes the research environment they create, the prerequisite skills they need to acquire, the roles and relationships they develop and the processes they use.

THE GLITTERING ARRAY

This chapter is about what person-centred researchers know and how they are, as a researcher, in their practice of developing new knowledge. The new knowledge created may or may not be specifically about person-centred health or social care or practice, but we argue, as a practice, it is always developed by paying attention to relational connectedness with participants

Person-Centred Healthcare Research, First Edition. Edited by Brendan McCormack, Sandra van Dulmen, Hilde Eide, Kirsti Skovdahl and Tom Eide.
© 2017 John Wiley & Sons Ltd. Published 2017 by John Wiley & Sons Ltd.

and co-researchers, the blending of different sources of knowledge and ways of knowing and creating supportive research environments and cultures. The beauty of doing person-centred research is that there is a glittering array of research worldviews and paradigms from which to choose. This choice is shaped by the person-centred outcomes we want to achieve, the questions we want to ask and the kind of research product we want to create. In this chapter, we open this treasure trove to show you three research worldviews within which person-centred research practice is usually located:

1. Practical.
2. Emancipatory.
3. Transformational.

We invite you to engage actively with the material we offer, so that this complex topic may become more personally meaningful to you.

Treasure troves are likely to look exciting, full of light and colour and jumbled. When novice researchers start looking at the treasure, they are often bedazzled and confused about the complex array of research paradigms and so they are blinded to the different bedrocks[1] that support these paradigms. Having been there ourselves, we know that if we pay attention to, and are systematic in, our examination of the bedrocks, we can begin to understand more clearly the differences between the philosophical assumptions of research worldviews, as well as, how the person-centred researcher can blend these assumptions systematically, as well as intuitively, to meet their purposes. We therefore present the bedrock assumptions in two ways, first through person-centred research narratives and then, later in the chapter, in a tabular form that builds on previous work by Angie and other colleagues.[2]

Discussing how we were going to write this chapter, we agreed that we would first explore our experiential knowing that McCormack and McCance's (2010) person-centred practice framework, developed originally in the context of health and social care, would be likely to work, with reconfiguration, for person-centred research practice. Therefore, we decided to write three person-centred research narratives located respectively in the *practical, emancipatory* and *transformational worldviews*, as well as test the supposition that our own research was underpinned by the same values and basic structure of the person-centred practice framework. Figure 3.1 shows our beginning epistemological and ontological framework for person-centred research. Figure 3.2, later in the chapter, shows how we have extended, deepened and refined our supposition through our writing-as-inquiry.

---

[1] The metaphor of bedrocks (research worldviews) supporting different research landscapes is described in more detail in Titchen and Horsfall (2011a).

[2] Included in the tables is a comparison with the assumptions of the quantitative *technical worldview*, within which many of us are first socialised as novice researchers. We contend that person-centred research is unlikely to be carried out within this worldview because relational connectedness and the blending of different sources of knowledge and ways of knowing are not encouraged. This does not mean, of course, that technical researchers who are undertaking studies concerned with measurement and quantification of person-centred health/social care practice, do not respect their subjects as persons or their self-determination to enter into or withdraw from the study at any time. However, technical researchers are unlikely to be concerned with creating the conditions for subjects' self-determination and involvement *within the research process itself* and for mutuality and reciprocity within their relationships with subjects. Indeed, such relationships and involvement would be detrimental to the rigour of work in this worldview. Nevertheless, we include the worldview in our tables to throw the other worldviews into relief and help crystallise your understanding of them.

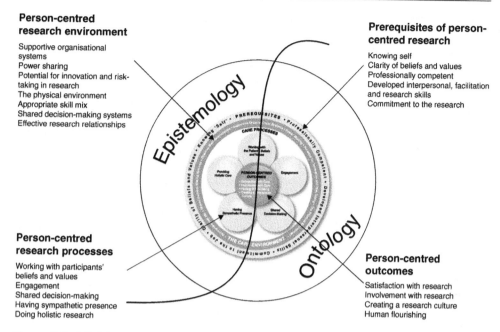

Person-centred research environment

Supportive organisational systems
Power sharing
Potential for innovation and risk-taking in research
The physical environment
Appropriate skill mix
Shared decision-making systems
Effective research relationships

Prerequisites of person-centred research

Knowing self
Clarity of beliefs and values
Professionally competent
Developed interpersonal, facilitation and research skills
Commitment to the research

Person-centred research processes

Working with participants' beliefs and values
Engagement
Shared decision-making
Having sympathetic presence
Doing holistic research

Person-centred outcomes

Satisfaction with research
Involvement with research
Creating a research culture
Human flourishing

Figure 3.1 Work in progress: epistemological and ontological framework for person-centred research. Source: Modified from McCormack and McCance (2010).

In Figure 3.1, you will notice the terms, 'epistemology' and 'ontology' in a new outer circle around McCormack and McCance's person-centred practice framework and a flowing line across the whole framework. This line symbolises the flowing, interactive, re-iterative relationship between the person-centred researcher's epistemology and ontology. Although they are separate entities, they are seamless and inextricably linked in practice because it is through our ontological practices that we are able to engage in knowledge creation using the epistemological assumptions of our worldview.

All you need to know before you read the narratives is that there are a number of research paradigms located within four major worldviews in research and practice development. Some of these paradigms are named in Appendix (Tables 3.A.1 and 3.A.2). If you are a novice researcher, we suggest that, later, you go through the meaning of all the tables carefully with your supervisor, an experienced research colleague or a peer group of PhD students or practitioner-researchers.

OPENING THE TREASURE TROVE

The first narrative by Stian is about his PhD research to understand the lived experience of people who abuse substances. He shows the epistemology and ontology of the *hermeneutic research paradigm*. As this paradigm is located in the *practical worldview*, the ultimate purpose of creating propositional (research/scholarly) knowledge is to develop understanding of the practice or the thing being investigated that is relevant to practice (hence the *practical* worldview). This new knowledge is then published and shared with others not involved in the research, so that they can use it in their practice. This worldview is underpinned by the bedrock of *idealism* that emphasises the ideas of participants as the determinant of social reality and human beings as having the ability to interpret their own and other's actions. Shaun, in his narrative, shows a very different research approach in which the findings are used by the co-researchers to change themselves or their practices within the research itself, as well as make it available for others to use subsequently. In his PhD, he co-inquired with nurse leaders into the nature and development of person-centred leadership and how they could free or eman-cipate themselves from inner and outer challenges that made being and becoming person-centred leaders difficult for them (including himself as facilitator/leader of the inquiry). His study is located in the *critical research paradigm* within the *emancipatory worldview*. In this worldview the ultimate purpose is again about developing propositional understanding, but understanding through taking action to bring about change and social justice. The bedrock of this worldview is *realism* that emphasises social structures and cultures as shaping practice and the determinants of social reality. Finally, Angie shares her ongoing co-critical-creative inquiry with PhD students and practice developers into how working in the *critical creativity paradigm* can be facilitated through critical–creative companionship. This paradigm is located in the *transformational worldview* and is concerned with developing propositional under-standing, bringing about change/transformation, social justice, as well as human flourishing.

You may notice how these three worldviews build on each other in an incremental 'yes and' relationship. It is important to remember that these worldviews are not separate entities and whilst it is good practice to locate a study in one worldview, researchers may decide to blend and meld assumptions from different worldviews. In which case, it is important to justify the combinations. The key point here is that it is important to understand the big picture when developing our methodologies so that we 'mix and match' assumptions appropriately.

We invite you now to hold the following questions in mind as you read the narratives. You will find some answers to these questions in Tables 3.A.1 and 3.A.2. In addition, you might like to apply these questions and the tables to your own research and/or compare Figure 3.1 with Figure 3.2 to check out our testing of the new epistemological and ontological framework.

1. How are language and meaning seen in this narrative?
2. What is the nature of the research question(s)?
3. What view of the person/world is evident in the writing?
4. What are the key person-centred values in the narrative?
5. How would you describe the relationship between the researcher and participants?
6. What kind of roles is the researcher adopting?
7. What is the ethical stance of the researcher?
8. What is the moral intent of this research?

STIAN'S NARRATIVE: ON APPROACHING RESEARCH FROM AN INTERPRETIVE HERMENEUTIC PARADIGM

In my research, I have been occupied by exploring and understanding the lived experiences of substance abuse, life-threatening overdoses and suicidal behaviour because there is a lack of knowledge based on an insider perspective that emerges from persons' lived experiences and *existence* (Biong, 2008; Biong, Karlsson and Svensson, 2008).

The key epistemological assumption of the interpretive hermeneutic paradigm is that such knowledge relies on multiple layers of interpretation; the teller when narrating, the researcher when analysing and the reader when reading, whilst the key underlying ontologi-cal assumption is that there is neither a single absolute truth of social reality nor one correct interpretation or understanding of human experiences and existence.

Social realities are assumed to be multiple and constructed, and our perceptions of them are mediated through a series of distorting lenses (Rolfe, 2006). In interpretive hermeneutic research, the researcher's pre-understanding forms an important and vital factor, and thus is not seen as a bias, rather as essential (Gadamer, 1989). Thus the researcher explicates this often tacit, *pre-understanding* or knowing and uses it in hearing and interpreting the shared meanings in the shared background of the participants' worlds. Some of the important *prerequisites of person-centred research* and attributes of the *research environment* in relation to interpretive hermeneutic research are, therefore, the researcher's knowing of oneself, and clarity of own beliefs and values (*reflexivity*). Reflexivity is defined as an attitude of the researcher, attending systematically to the context of knowledge co-construction, especially in relation to the effect on the researcher, at every step of the research process (Malterud, 2001).

When I started my research in 2004, in Norway the medical model of addiction had taken over a more social model (Sælør and Biong, 2011). However, I did not want to use a medical discourse. Therefore, I decided not to use language or ask questions that referred to persons as 'sick', but would instead probe for more details and reflections about their daily lives and own views on their *existence*, in order to affirm them as active and creative agents in their lives (*existentialism*). Whilst being aware of the insidious effect of the medical model discourse within public health on me and on people with substance abuse, I wanted my interpretive research to give voice to other ways of understanding highly stigmatised social practices. Theoretically, I had been mainly informed by the medical understanding taught at the nursing school (which in fact was very little at all). Consequently, my public health practice was mainly concerned with explaining and handling risk factors and prevention. When my research career began in 2001, the concept of 'new' public health presented a different view of public health as a complex interplay of individual, cultural and societal factors, making more *existential philosophical approaches* possible. Introduced to these new ideas, my pre-understanding was challenged and broadened to include holistic *understanding and meaning-making* systems. This was *reflexivity* in action.

Interpretive hermeneutic research can be conducted solely by a researcher or in co-inquiry relationships (Beresford, 2003). In my study, participants were partially co-inquirers as I provided opportunities to co-construct different kinds of knowledge of substance abuse and suicidal behaviour. These were *ideographic knowledge* about the individual participants' subjective meaning based on the interaction between the participants and society (*idealism*) and *scientific knowledge* from the evaluation of my work by a community of researchers. However, I was the one who chose the topic of research, developed the research protocol and formulated the research questions. This might not be fully in line with the power sharing and shared decision-making of person-centred research environments, but choosing a narrative approach enabled participants in my study to cooperate in self-determined ways. For example, while telling his story one participant asked me, 'How deep will you go into this matter?', demonstrating his power to choose to proceed with further details or not.

To gain a deeper understanding of the *meaning* (existence) of substance abuse, life threatening overdoses and suicidal behaviour (Ricoeur, 1976), I chose a narrative approach in which facilitation of individual research interviews became a way of *illuminating understanding and meaning* (Polkinghorne, 1988). My scientific training had equipped me to conduct unstructured interviews, with one opening question, around which the participants then could associate freely. The intention was that through the *person-centred research processes* of engaging and working together, during the interviews, participants should be able to share their experiences and to tell what they wanted to tell about their experiences to an active and open-minded listener. Therefore, interviews became more of a conversation between two persons who were working in *partnership*.

As the researcher–participant relationship is deemed a significant part of the *person-centred research processes*, but our time together was relatively short, I tried to *connect* us by creating a climate that was as relaxed, calm, psychologically safe and trusting as possible. Usually we started with a cup of coffee and informal chat for half-an-hour or so before we began the interview. Sometimes participants initiated the *creation of this environment*, for example, one participant prepared dinner for us and another arranged a day-trip to the area where he lived.

Interpretive hermeneutic research views scientific knowledge as co-constructed in social processes of several levels of interpretation (Ricoeur, 1976; Beresford, 2003). The use of qualitative research interviews in person-centred research invites persons to speak about their perceived world in their own words, working out and articulating their previously tacit pre-understanding of what happened. With the use of *language*, stories about lived experiences are constructed in broader historical, social and cultural contexts (Ricoeur, 1976). Open-ended, unstructured narrative interviewing allows narrators to tell what they want to tell, interpret their earlier experiences and, thus, obtain meaning and identities. Both the narrator and the listener become active participants in the *co-construction* and *co-production* of the understanding and meaning of the lived experience. As an active listener, not only did I listen to what was said, I was also attentive to what was happening in terms of power and emotions. Given the very personal topic of the interviews, I was mindful of respecting participants' integrity and dignity and not doing harm or making them feel insecure. I was aware that there may be themes into which I should not probe too deeply.

The interviews lasted between one-and-half and two hours and ended by asking if there was something more the participant would like to add. We then sat and talked a little about how it had been to participate and how the participant felt at that moment. As part of the *person-centred research process*, I asked if some kind of (psychosocial) follow-up support was needed. This support had been prepared because I did not want to expose the participants to more stress than necessary. To my knowledge, several of the participants received planned and closer follow-up from staff after the interview due to the reactions they had experienced. I also agreed to contact each person after a short while to hear how they were doing.

The potential social- and self-stigma linked to the phenomena in my investigation triggered my reflexivity on how I thought and acted towards the participants (Goffman, 1963). However, they seemed to share their experiences willingly, and several shared how no-one had talked to them about their experiences and thoughts about what had happened in this way before. All said that they had been motivated to participate because 'hopefully, this can help others'. I was authentic, quiet and attended to my listening, probing and showing an interest in their telling. I see this today as balancing innovation and risk taking in the *person-centred research environment*. In contrast to the critical and critical creativity paradigms, collaboration with the participants might end after the interview with participants in interpretive hermeneutic research. However, it is important to bear in mind that full co-inquiry or degrees of it, for the purpose of gaining understanding, is still possible within this paradigm, especially when practitioners are researching their own practices together.

SHAUN'S NARRATIVE: ON APPROACHING RESEARCH FROM A CRITICAL PARADIGM

Approaching research in a person-centred way, I created a philosophical framework for my doctoral study that explored and developed person-centred leadership through critical participatory action research (Cardiff, 2014). My framework pulls assumptions from the *emancipatory* (critical realism, critical social science) and *transformational* (critical creativity) *worldviews*.

Unlike the constructivist and hermeneutic paradigms, I believe that *social reality* is mind independent, complex and deeply layered (stratified), i.e. it has an empirical, actual and real domain. Unobservable mechanisms/powers in the real domain have the potential of generating events in time and space in the actual domain that can be observed in the real domain (Danermark *et al.*, 2002). Mechanisms/powers are viewed as always present, but can remain dormant, be activated or counteracted by other mechanisms/powers.

Like the constructivist and hermeneutic paradigms, people's observations and interpretations of social contexts and events are the primary source of access to understanding *social reality*. In addition, social experimentation and critical dialogue is essential for co-creating robust knowledge of the world we live in. However, in line with the transformational worldview, I also believe that dialogue through the spoken word alone can be restricting. Both a person's vocabulary and cognitive rationalisation (thinking: 'I can't/don't need to say that') can limit what they share. *Embodied knowledge* may not reach conscious thought and so not be verbalised. The use of creative expression helps overcome these restrictions. I simplify this complex interplay of layers and co-production of knowledge with the expression 'what we (as distinct persons) perceive is not necessarily all that there is'. Also, a mechanism of particular interest to critical social scientists is how the manifestation of power can enhance and/or inhibit the self-actualisation, empowerment and wellbeing of people. To illustrate these assumptions in action I start with one event I observed and offer a plausible explanation for its manifestation. I then discuss how attentiveness to person-centred values emancipated and transformed both participants' and my own being.

In my PhD study I observed a newly qualified staff nurse happily resigning from the nursing unit, which surprised me as she had previously expressed being happy and not wanting, or intending to leave the unit. However, other events had taken place beforehand, in a different time and space. During appraisals of her integration into the unit people had expressed how they liked her as a person, but were concerned about the rate she was developing the required professional competences. It was placing a burden on staff and there were concerns about possible implications for patient safety and quality of care. The nurse had a year-long contract, which offered the charge nurse a structure and power mechanism for the enforced departure of the staff nurse from the unit. This mechanism was not activated and while the event of her leaving the unit was the same, she left happily of her own free will. This raised the question of what different mechanism/power had been activated.

I had been facilitating critical and creative *reflective* inquiries (Cardiff, 2012) into participant leadership. The staff nurse who was failing to develop the competences needed to work effectively on the unit was one inquiry. During the inquiry, the leaders analysed the situation, leader behaviour, possible actions and possible consequences. The key question was 'what is the right thing to do?' The use of tableau vivant (a creative expression of a narrative using real people and materials within the context) offered participants a means of non-verbally communicating *(pre)conscious interpretations and understandings* of the narrative. This was followed by *critical dialogue* on interpretations of each tableau vivant. Facilitating consideration of both bodily and visual perceptions, values and beliefs underlying interpretations and understandings, revealed conflicts between intentions and expectations, as well as possible alternative actions more congruent with person-centred values. The conclusion was that realisation of the previously agreed aim of a person-centred leader (enabling staff to 'come into their own', i.e. experience self-actualisation, empowerment and wellbeing) required a different course of action. The charge nurse consequently discussed the staff nurse's wellbeing, coping and ambitions with her. Collaboratively, they explored opportunities of employment elsewhere and the staff nurse secured a job in a long-term care facility, which she was very happy with. This event demonstrates that we (the nurse leader co-inquirers and myself) had created conditions for leader *reflexivity*, which in this case, led to a change in leadership practice that enhanced rather than damaged a staff nurse's personhood.

As stated in a constructivist paradigm, *practical knowledge* is produced through human relating and agency. Like the hermeneutic paradigm, the critical paradigm accepts that multiple perceptions and understandings can co-exist, so knowledge should be co-created. These paradigms share the assumption that co-creation starts with our experience of events and that there is potential to emancipate and/or transform values, beliefs, relating and agency. However, it is only in the critical and transformational paradigms that there is an intention to *facilitate emancipation and transformation*. There is an assumption that this in turn can produce different social structures, conventions and practices that will influence future agency and relating, as well as flourishing in the critical creativity paradigm.

We are contextual and historical beings who try to understand observed reality, but are restricted by the values and beliefs, concepts and theoretical frameworks we (as individuals and as a collective) hold at any moment in time (Fay, 1987). For this reason, creating psychologically critical and creative communicative spaces is a means to foster *authentic engagement* and robust inquiry into these restrictions. The inquiry sessions above, as well as the post-observation interviews I conducted, are examples of such spaces. However, if we fear reprisal for what we share in these communal spaces, we may be unable to engage authentically or robustly because we refrain from contributing knowledge and interpretations for *contestation and debate*, or we may distance ourselves from the dialogue. To achieve (psychological) safety so participants would feel comfortable in sharing and analysing their lived experiences, I needed to observe and reflect on my own being in relation with them.

By the end of the study, both the participants and I discovered that *relational connectedness* was key to achieving a leader/facilitator goal of enabling self and others to 'come into their own'. We found it requires characteristics such as being authentically other-centred and caring, knowing self, being reflexive, patient, optimistic and open, as well as a willingness to show vulnerability. Knowing the other and achieving a sense of connectedness entailed engaging in processes of sensing (using one's senses to assess the other person's wellbeing at that moment in time); contextualising (seeing and understanding them as a person embedded within multiple influencing contexts); balancing (considering needs of other and self); presencing (being and thinking with the other person), and communing (action-oriented dialogue). Using the information gathered by engaging in these processes enabled us to determine a response (stance) that could foster 'coming into own'. Self-determination, mutuality and reciprocity were enhanced. Participant evaluations revealed that by working towards relational connectedness, including them in the design of the study and enabling participation in research activities, encouraged them to commit time and energy for three years in fieldwork and subsequent member checking of the thesis.

As active beings we also co-construct social contexts, including the research context (Fay, 1987). Engaging in this action research study on person-centred leadership emancipated me from objectivity and researcher distance values acquired when I undertook a quantitative study in the *technical worldview* for my master's degree, and transformed my being as a researcher. I came to appreciate how as traditional and embedded beings we often uncritically reproduce social structures, conventions and practices, but as active beings we also possess the potential to transform them. Through (supported) reflexivity I was able to change or adjust my research plans/activities so as to meet participant needs without jeopardising the quality of data gathering or analysis. For instance, we had agreed for participant leaders to facilitate storytelling sessions with staff, but they kept postponing the start date. I could have appealed to their sense of responsibility towards agreed plans and/or manipulated them into starting before they felt ready. However, this would not have respected their rights to self-determination and could have potentially damaged our relational connectedness. They valued the fact that I 'moved with them'. They remained engaged, storytelling sessions did commence (later than expected) and data gathering was achieved.

In conclusion, my experience is that social scientists working within an emancipatory worldview may need to review their philosophical and ethical beliefs as they facilitate critical co-inquiry from a person-centred paradigm based on values of respect, self-determination, mutuality and reciprocity. I believe that social research should begin with human perceptions of the empirical and actual layers and that knowledge should be co-produced. This requires researcher reflexivity as our own being can potentially (dis)enable knowledge co-creation and co-production. As a person-centred researcher I believe we should work towards relational connectedness and the creation of psychologically safe, critical and creative communicative spaces from which emancipatory and transformative action can emerge. This entails conscious and intentional movement through different levels of engagement with participants and the context. The aim should be for each person to feel acknowledged and valued as a distinct individual with a valuable contribution to make in the co-production of robust knowledge.

ANGIE'S NARRATIVE: ON APPROACHING RESEARCH FROM THE CRITICAL CREATIVITY PARADIGM

In my narrative, I focus primarily on epistemological and ontological assumptions that differentiate the *transformational worldview* from the practical and critical worldviews. I will share something of an international co-inquiry that I am currently engaged in as a critical–creative companion to a social worker, a PhD student and two practice developers in nursing. We are all practitioner-researchers using and investigating how we use critical creativity in our practices and we each have our own inquiry questions. Building on my critical companionship research, my questions are 'How do I do critical–creative companionship to help co-inquirers answer their own inquiry questions?' (*epistemological question*) and 'What does it mean to be a critical–creative companion?' (*ontological question*).

Critical creativity is a paradigmatic synthesis in which the assumptions of the critical paradigm are blended and balanced with, and connected and attuned to, creative, ecological and spiritual traditions, ancient wisdom, wisdom of the body, beauty, spirituality, and the natural world for the purpose of human flourishing. Human flourishing focuses on maximising individuals' achievement of their potential for growth and development as they change the circumstances and relations of their lives. People are helped to flourish (i.e. grow, develop, thrive) during the change experience in addition to an intended outcome of well-being for the beneficiaries of the work (McCormack and Titchen, 2006; Titchen and McCormack, 2008, 2010; McCormack and Titchen, 2014, 2015).

With my co-inquirers, my intention has been to act as the facilitator of the space and activity of our first retreat together and, thereafter, for us to co-facilitate, so that: (a) we are creating a *person-centred research environment*, in terms of sharing and circulating power and decision-making, providing potential and physical environments for innovation and risk-taking, as well as developing effective research relationships; and (b) co-inquirers *contribute to the design of the retreat* and have the opportunity to *practise the facilitation and research skills and processes*. We have found that being together in retreat, especially over a weekend in each other's home, sharing the preparation of food and a bottle of wine, has enabled the development of really close, trusting, *person-centred relationships* and friendships. This *connecting together as people* has been vital in my experience of doing person-centred research in both the interpretive and critical paradigms, but this communal living for a short period takes it a step further.

My role is the lead inquirer and, in this role, I adopt a facilitative, person-centred relationship with co-inquirers. This is necessary because they are not cognizant with the philosophical, theoretical and methodological aspects of critical creativity research and accessing, working with and blending the multiple sources of wisdom, pre-reflective knowledge and ways of knowing. Therefore, I am often helping my co-inquirers to *create research and practice development environments and cultures* that are open to these unusual ways of knowing, doing, being and becoming, and developing the skills to do so, and to do the research.

I support co-inquirers' exploration of critical creativity by sharing the part played by the bedrocks of *idealism* (emphasis on participants' ideas about social reality, i.e. what people consciously know), *existentialism* (emphasis on the place of pre-reflective knowing, doing, being and becoming in developing knowledge and bringing about transformation), *hermeneutics* (the study of understanding through processes akin to creating or appreciating a piece of art) and *realism* (overcoming structures and cultures that challenge the delivery of person-centred practice). I explain that critical creativity adds the bedrocks of *metaphysics* (the non-empirical study of the nature of existence, e.g. through myths, imagination, artistic expression) and *aesthetics* (the study of beauty). This synthesis forms the philosophical bedrock of critical creativity. However, I make it clear that they may not draw on all the bedrocks or all their assumptions in one study! Making sense of this mix before they design their research and choose their assumptions is complex and people need help.

But I don't start with a treatise! Rather, I provide co-inquirers with the experience of the bedrock synthesis in action, usually on retreat in beautiful countryside[3]. I intentionally role-model the philosophical assumptions and I articulate my practical and theoretical know-how, either in the moment or as near it as possible. For example, guided by the assumption of a *holistic view of the person and the world*, within critical creativity, the world extends beyond the life and social worlds to include the natural world. I provide the conditions and strategies to enable co-inquirers to respect deeply, connect with, and immerse themselves in, nature and the ecology of our planet. This immersion is the *primary point of access to reality*. This is why our retreats partially happen by rivers, fields, rocky places and woods and why we work with the whole of ourselves – body, soul, mind, heart, imagination, creativity and ancient wisdom to provide material for *artistic and cognitive critique* in both the development and sharing of new knowledge (see Titchen and Horsfall, 2011b; McCormack and Titchen, 2015). When we open up all our physical senses and imagination to this source, we fall into the beauty, mystery and energy of the natural world and see the messages there for us. We might frame our inner worlds, thoughts and understanding in the landscape. Let me give you an example.

Lorna is a PhD student embarking on a study of human flourishing in healthcare. She has been struggling with getting to grips with the philosophical underpinnings of research.

---

[3] Sometimes this is not possible and we work equally effectively in a hospital garden or city park. Or if this is not possible, we bring natural objects indoors, such as stones or flowers or work with images from nature (e.g. photos or the inner eye).

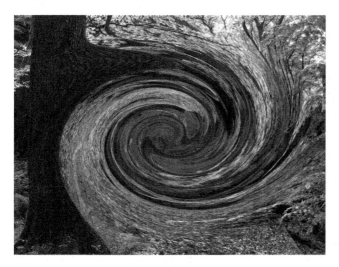

Flying through spaces in the imagination provides powerful images of understanding and insight. This was my experience when I undertook a creative visioning exercise in the beautiful Cotswolds with Angie ... We are using critical creativity approaches to increase my understanding of how the paradigm of critical creativity can support and hold my methodological and philosophical assumptions together. I also wanted to distinguish the different research landscapes or paradigms that are supported by the different bedrocks...

Leaning against an ancient tree, we began the exercise by closing our eyes. Creative visioning was instantly appealing to me. I noticed that as soon as I closed my eyes and Angie started talking me through the journey, I linked almost instantly with my imagination. I can describe it as having one foot in the present and being aware of my body in relation to where I was sitting, and one foot in an imaginary landscape. I was climbing on the back of a huge heron and flying away from the tree ... away into the distance to a technical research landscape. Guiding me through the journey, Angie asked me to experience the flight imaginatively with all my senses.

When I had reached the technical bedrock, she asked me what I could see, smell, hear, taste and touch ... Climbing back on the heron, I was flying away to another landscape – a transformational bedrock and landscape garden. The contrast to the technical image was huge...

This visioning exercise enabled me to picture in a deep and powerful way what my research philosophical underpinnings might look like. Also, at a very profound level, I understood the significance of whole body engagement and bringing in creative and ancient ways of knowing, as well as rational, cognitive ways of knowing, so that we can bring the whole of ourselves to our research and practice development. This consolidated, for me, my decision that critical creativity with its focus on transformation and human flourishing was congruent with virtue ethics and would, therefore, be my research paradigm. (Source: Peelo-Kilroe, 2014.)

Becoming a transformational researcher requires deep work *to know oneself* and to develop the skills of helping others to become co-inquirers on their transformation of self, teams, workplaces and organisation. It requires opening ourselves to ways of *knowing, doing, being and becoming* and ways of *languaging and making meaning* that we may be unfamiliar with. For example, my co-inquirers have opened their hearts to the idea that spirituality in the critical creativity paradigm is not connected with religion or doctrine of any kind. It is about working at the edge of the known in search of meaning through connecting with our metaphysical Greater Self and the wisdom of nature, the universe and all the ancient peoples that have lived on this planet and who have been much closer to nature than our generations have been. We have found that intentionally opening up our hearts creates the conditions for reciprocal loving kindness, compassion and grace to flow, especially through times of inner and outer turbulence, and enables us to flourish through the process of the research. We have also learned that letting go of ego and being attached to outcome is vital in person-centred research and in enabling all involved to flourish.

A BEGINNING EPISTEMOLOGICAL AND ONTOLOGICAL FRAMEWORK FOR PERSON-CENTRED RESEARCH

In our narratives, we have pointed out what we think are examples of the attributes and basic structure of the new, but borrowed person-centred research framework (Figure 3.1). After a careful analysis of the narratives to seek for commonalities across the worldviews, several environmental conditions, prerequisites, research processes and an outcome emerged which transcend the particular worldviews within which the researcher works. Broadly, these are:

- *Person-centred research environment*: person-centred researchers are aware of contextual influences on the relationships they have with participants, their own being and the research process;
- *Pre-requisites for person-centred research*: a collection of researcher attributes were identified in the narratives, the most prominent/important of which is reflexivity. A reflexive researcher should be able to articulate and reflect on their personal values, beliefs and needs (being and becoming) and from this act with a moral intention of doing 'good';
- *Person-centred research processes*: a number of processes characterise person-centred research, all of which contribute to the creation of (virtual) safe, critical and creative communicative spaces; and
- *Person-centred research outcomes:* participant and researcher wellbeing/flourishing during (and after) the research period.

The specifics are set out in Figure 3.2.

Through our writing we have shown similarities and differences in the three sets of person-centred, epistemological and ontological assumptions underpinning the practical, emancipatory and transformational worldviews. We have illustrated how these three sets are interdependent and intertwined and how the skilled person-centred researcher is able to occupy all three spaces either simultaneously or flow seamlessly from one space to another in the moment. This multilayered, dynamic skill is symbolised by the curved line that you might like to imagine as spinning to blend and meld the three sets of assumptions.

Tables 3.A.1 and 3.A.2 set out, in broad continua, the epistemological and ontological assumptions that person-centred researchers might consider. They were developed originally from Angie's doctoral research, refined and elaborated on with others (Titchen and Hobson, 2005; Titchen and Higgs, 2007) and set in the context of action research (Titchen, 2015). They have now been broadened and refined again in the context of person-centred research.

As we move from left to right of the tables, the continua give person-centred researchers a much wider palette of assumptions to blend and meld when meeting the challenges of living the person-centred values of respect, reciprocity, mutuality and self-determination in every aspect of the research. For example, in the interpretive hermeneutic paradigm, Stian's ontological assumptions about the *determinant of reality* shaped his interview approach with participants and his subsequent knowledge development. To get at people's lived experiences, he needed to access what they knew both consciously (in the mind) and unconsciously (through the body and being immersed in their life and social worlds), so he drew on the assumptions of both *practical worldviews* for his primary sources of access. So did Shaun and Angie, but Shaun added the assumption that what people know through connections with each other

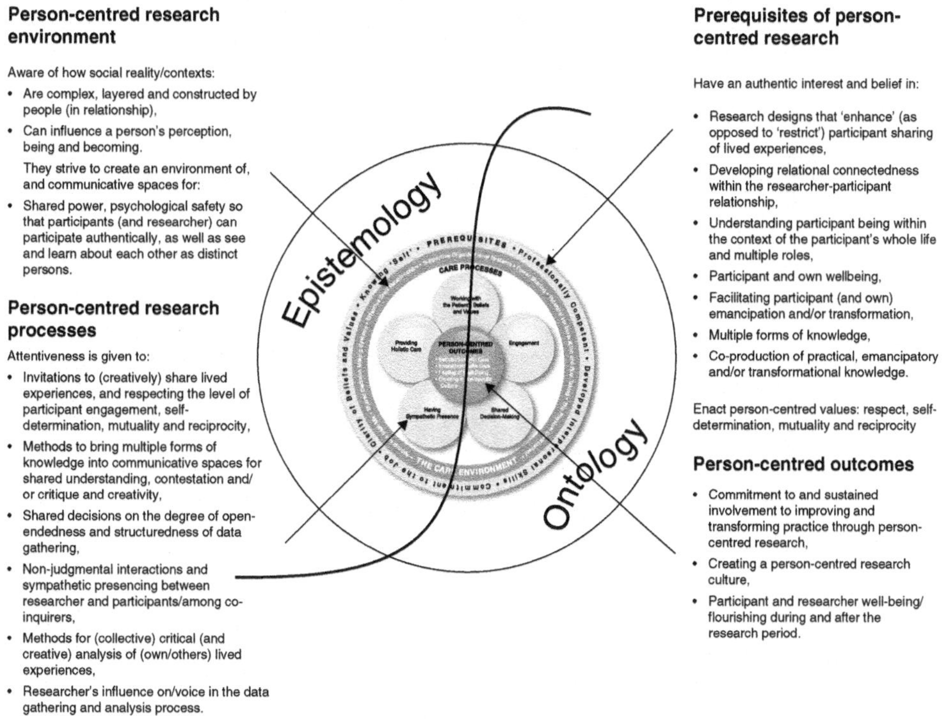
Person-centred research environment
Aware of how social reality/contexts:
• Are complex, layered and constructed by people (in relationship),
• Can influence a person's perception, being and becoming.
They strive to create an environment of, and communicative spaces for:
• Shared power, psychological safety so that participants (and researcher) can participate authentically, as well as see and learn about each other as distinct persons.
Person-centred research processes
Attentiveness is given to:
• Invitations to (creatively) share lived experiences, and respecting the level of participant engagement, self-determination, mutuality and reciprocity,
• Methods to bring multiple forms of knowledge into communicative spaces for shared understanding, contestation and/ or critique and creativity,
• Shared decisions on the degree of open-endedness and structuredness of data gathering,
• Non-judgmental interactions and sympathetic presencing between researcher and participants/among co-inquirers,
• Methods for (collective) critical (and creative) analysis of (own/others) lived experiences,
• Researcher's influence on/voice in the data gathering and analysis process.
Epistemology
Ontology
PREREQUISITES
CARE PROCESSES
THE CARE ENVIRONMENT
PERSON-CENTRED OUTCOMES
Prerequisites of person-centred research
Have an authentic interest and belief in:
• Research designs that 'enhance' (as opposed to 'restrict') participant sharing of lived experiences,
• Developing relational connectedness within the researcher-participant relationship,
• Understanding participant being within the context of the participant's whole life and multiple roles,
• Participant and own wellbeing,
• Facilitating participant (and own) emancipation and/or transformation,
• Multiple forms of knowledge,
• Co-production of practical, emancipatory and/or transformational knowledge.
Enact person-centred values: respect, self-determination, mutuality and reciprocity
Person-centred outcomes
• Commitment to and sustained involvement to improving and transforming practice through person-centred research,
• Creating a person-centred research culture,
• Participant and researcher well-being/ flourishing during and after the research period.

Figure 3.2 Epistemological and ontological framework for person-centred research. Source: Modified from McCormack and McCance (2010).

(social practice) is another primary point of access. This had different implications for knowledge development, so in partnership with his co-researchers, Shaun used a creative hermeneutic approach that included use of the body and artistic expression to make sense and meaning. Knowledge development occurred through critique and reflectivity. In addition, Angie melded and blended these primary sources of access with what people know through connection with the natural world, ecosystems linked to ancient wisdom and spiritual traditions. So, in her inquiry, knowledge development is occurring by combining the knowing surfaced through this non-empirical point of access with mental representation and knowing in and through body, practice and social practices. This occurs through artistic and cognitive critique.

CONCLUSION

A tentative new epistemological and ontological framework for person-centred research has been developed in this chapter from studies only in three paradigms through inquiry-by-writing. However, as it has built on many years of rigorous philosophical, theoretical and methodological work by Brendan McCormack, Tanya McCance and Angie Titchen, separately and together, and as we feel from our personal research experience and knowledge of the constructivist, interpretive and 8th moment paradigms, we conclude that this framework is probably more widely relevant. This is for you and others to determine! Moreover, we propose that the fundamental, person-centred values of respect, reciprocity, mutuality and self-determination are all present in the practical, emancipatory and transformational worldviews, but they might be present to different degrees according to the worldview purpose.

APPENDIX

Table 3.A.1 Philosophical (i.e. epistemological and ontological) assumptions of the four worldviews.

Worldview	Technical	Practical (a)	Practical (b)	Emancipatory	Transformational
Philosophical stance	Empiricism/rationalism	Idealism	Existentialism	++[a] Realism	+++[b] Metaphysics/aesthetics
Research paradigm	Empirico-analytical	Interpretive Constructivist	Interpretive Hermeneutic	Critical	Critical creativity New paradigm/8th moment
Determinants of reality	Reality is mind independent, i.e. exists independent of human perception. Sense data is the only source of access to knowledge of the world (objectivity is key)	Reality is not mind independent, i.e. linked to human perception. What people know consciously (mental representations) is the primary source of access to knowledge of the world	Reality is not mind independent, i.e. linked to human perception. What people know in and through their bodies and practices (pre-reflective, shared meanings in shared background practices) is primary point of access	++[b] Reality is layered. There is a reality independent of the human mind, but we can only comprehend/study that which we perceive at the moment and in the context of what we already know. What people know through connections with each other (social practice) is the primary point of access	+++[b] What people know through connection with the natural world, ecosystems linked to ancient wisdom and spiritual traditions is the primary point of access. Knowing surfaced through this non-empirical point of access is then combined with mental representation and knowing in and through body, practice and social practices. This occurs through artistic and cognitive critique

	Instrumental knowledge	Practical knowledge	+^c Practical knowledge	++^a Emancipatory/ transformative knowledge	+++ ^b Transformational knowledge
Knowledge; ways of knowing that researcher seeks to access from participants and then develop into propositional knowledge	*Explanation/prediction* Observation of cause and effect, measurement, description	*Understanding* Practice wisdom, experiential, ethical/moral, personal, aesthetic, spiritual, intuitive knowledges that have mental representation (Habermas, 1984)	*Understanding* Practice wisdom, experiential knowledge, imagination, dreams, multiple intelligences, ethical/moral, personal, aesthetic, spiritual, intuitive, creative, embodied and othered (e.g. people with dementia, learning disabilities) ways of knowing that have no mental representation (Polanyi, 1951)	++^a *Critique/reflectivity /reflexivity* Our perception of the world is expressed in language. As a storytelling species, narrative knowledge can be added. 'Knowing that, knowing how and knowing what it is like' can be co-constructed and is influenced/limited by existent conceptualisations, social structures, conventions and practices. When critically derived, knowledge has the potential to transform social reality (which in turn will influence future), knowledge becomes ever evolving. But in an ever changing world, knowledge is transitive/ fallible. There are different valid perspectives of reality	++^a *Critical–creative critique and appreciation* More focus on creative imagination, creative ways of knowing and multiple intelligences in making connections with ancient wisdom and wonders and mysteries of the natural world and universe (of which people are a part)
Language and meaning	Language and meaning seen as objective entities	Language and meaning are constructed in social relationships	Language and meaning (through words, body and creative expression) refer to/are related to social context and social practice (and shared meanings in background practices). They are as 'real' as the physical, but can be conceptualised by means of different concepts and frameworks	++^a The way we perceive and live in the world may be expressed differently by individuals/groups through language and so dialogue is needed to find shared understandings/meaning that offer plausible descriptions and explanations	+++^b Creative expression, framing and drawing from nature and our connection with it

(Continued)

Table 3.A.1 (Continued)

Worldview	Technical	Practical (a)	Practical (b)	Emancipatory	Transformational
Nature of research questions	Instrumental research questions only	Epistemological research questions only	Ontological research questions only	Epistemological and/or ontological research questions	+[c]
View of the person/world	Individuality of persons is not the focus Person is seen as separate from the world (subject/object split)	Individuality of person +[c]	Being-in-the-world There is no separation of subject and object. The person is part of, and immersed in, the world	++[a] Welfare of the person/community is the focus ++[a] Person is seen as embedded in and (co)creator of social world (structures, conventions and practices), but separate from physical world	+++[b] Transformation and flourishing of the person and community ++[a] The person is connected with and immersed in the natural world
	The person is a provider of sense data in terms of their experience of the tool/intervention/concept being developed and tested; or an instrument to carry out action (in action-oriented research)	The person is a provider of data about his/her experience of the phenomenon being studied by the researcher, unless participants are co-researchers. Holistic view of person may be present, but focus is on what the person knows about the whole self, but only with their mind	+[c] Co-creation and co-construction	++[a]	+++[b]
			Holistic view of person and focus on what the heart, body, soul/spirit knows	++[a] Holistic view of person may be present, but focus is on what person knows about social structures, conventions and practices	+++[b] Holistic view of person includes the soul, mind, imagination, creativity embodied in the human spirit. Open to all ways of being

[a] ++ means 'in addition to the content of the previous **two** boxes in this row' (idealism + existentialism/aesthetics) in any combination.
[b] +++ means 'in addition to the content of the previous **three** boxes in this row' (idealism + existentialism/aesthetics + realism) in any combination.
[c] + means 'in addition to the content of the **previous** box in this row'.

Table 3.A.2 Implications of philosophical assumptions for person-centred research(er).

Worldview	Technical	Practical (a)	Practical (b)	Emancipatory	Transformational
Philosophical stance	Empiricism/rationalism	Idealism	Existentialism	++[a] Realism	+++[b] Metaphysics/aesthetics
Research paradigm	Empirico-analytical	Interpretive Constructivist	Interpretive Hermeneutic	Critical	Critical creativity New paradigm/8th moment
Key person-centred values	Researcher respects a person's integrity, dignity, security and values their contribution	+[c] Could also include mutuality and reciprocity, so honouring self-determination and cooperation	++[a]	+++[b] Social justice, mutuality, reciprocity, self-determination, cooperation, collaboration, inclusion and participation are always valued	++++[d] Human flourishing for all involved as end and means of research is valued
Relationships	Researcher–participant relationship is not deemed significant to research	Researcher–participant relationship is deemed a significant part of the research process in terms of acknowledging how the researcher can influence findings	+[c]	++[a] Researchers, participants and co-researchers include observation of self. Facilitator creating conditions for social justice	+++[b] Facilitator creating the conditions for human flourishing of all involved
	Relational distance is maintained in order to meet objectivity criteria	Engagement is aimed at building trust so that participants will share. Participants may be co-researchers, but it is their constructions of reality that are the object of study, not the researcher's. Researcher is aware and explicit about own pre-understandings and own personal, theoretical understandings and attempts to 'bracket' these in order to let participant data speak for itself	Engagement aimed at enabling 'fusion of horizons' reflexively. Researcher is aware and explicit in particular about how own pre-understandings (prejudices) can influence interpretations of texts, but not attempt to bracket them, rather seeks to develop reflexively 'a fusion of horizons' of others' and own perspectives. Unlikely to draw on theoretical understandings from literature	+[c] Researcher engages with participants, working towards relational connectedness ++[a] Researcher explicitly uses own and participant knowledge to co-construct/co-produce knowledge	++[a] Reciprocal loving kindness and grace +++[b] Bringing whole self as a person (mind, heart, body, soul) into relationships

(Continued)

Table 3.A.2 (Continued)

Worldview	Technical	Practical (a)	Practical (b)	Emancipatory	Transformational
Roles	Uninvolved, detached from participants and outcomes observer/researcher	Involved, connected to participants but detached (from outcome) observer/researcher	+[c]	Facilitator of action, observation and reflection on whether others'/own actions achieved intended outcome(s)	+[c] Facilitator of co-inquirers to enable use whole of selves in research
Ethics	Kantian ethics	+[c] Ethics of care when participants are cooperating in the research (dignity, respect, safety)	++[a]	++[a] Relational ethics. Participants may choose not to remain anonymous (reciprocity, mutuality, trust)	+[c]
Moral intent	Explain and predict social practices	Describe social practices	+[c] Interpret social practices	++[a] Change social practices Empowerment and emancipation (social justice)	+++[b] Transformation of self and others (if they so wish); human flourishing

[a] ++ means 'in addition to the content of the previous **two** boxes in this row' (idealism + existentialism/aesthetics) in any combination.

[b] +++ means 'in addition to the content of the previous **three** boxes in this row' (idealism + existentialism/aesthetics + realism) in any combination.

[c] + means 'in addition to the content of the **previous** box in this row'.

[d] ++++ means 'in addition to the content of the previous **four** boxes in this row'.

REFERENCES

Beresford, P. (2003) User involvement in research: exploring the challenges. *Nursing Times Research*, **8**, 36–46.

Biong, S. (2008) *Between Death as Escape and the Dream of Life. Psychosocial Dimensions of Health in Young Men Living With Substance Abuse and Suicidal Behaviour*. Doctoral thesis. Nordic School of Public Health, Göteborg.

Biong, S., Karlsson, B. and Svensson, T. (2008) Metaphors of a shifting sense of self in men recovering from substance abuse and suicidal behavior. *Journal of Psychosocial Nursing*, **40**, 35–41.

Bullock, A. and Trombley, S. (Eds) (2000) *The New Fontana Dictionary of Modern Thought*, 3rd edn. Harper Collins, London.

Cardiff, S. (2012) Critical and creative reflective inquiry: surfacing narratives to enable learning and inform action. *Educational Action Research: An International Journal*, **20**, 605–622.

Cardiff, S. (2014) *Person-Centred Leadership: A Critical Participatory Action Research Study Exploring and Developing a New Style of (Clinical) Nurse Leadership*. PhD Thesis. University of Ulster, Belfast.

Danermark, B., Ekström, M., Jakobsen, L. and Karlsson, J. (2002) *Explaining Society: Critical Realism in the Social Sciences*. Routledge, Oxon.

Fay, B. (1987) *Critical Social Science: Liberation and its Limits*. Cornell University Press, New York.

Gadamer, H.-G. (1989) *Truth and Method*. Sheed & Ward, London.

Goffman, E. (1963) *Stigma, Notes on the Management of Spoiled Identity*. Prentice Hall, Upper Saddle River.

Guba, E.G. (1990) *The Paradigm Dialog*. Sage, Newbury Park.

Habermas, J. (1984) *Theory of Communicative Action, Volume One: Reason and the Rationalization of Society*, Translated by Thomas A. McCarthy. Beacon Press, Boston.

Malterud, K. (2001) Qualitative research: standards, challenges, and guidelines. *Lancet*, **358**, 483–488.

McCormack, B. and McCance, T. (2010) *Person-Centred Nursing: Theory and Practice*. Wiley Blackwell, Oxford.

McCormack, B. and Titchen, A. (2006) Critical creativity: melding, exploding, blending. *Educational Action Research: An International Journal*, **14**, 239–266.

McCormack, B. and Titchen, A. (2014) No beginning, no end: an ecology of human flourishing. *International Practice Development Journal*, **4**. http://www.fons.org/library/journal/volume4-issue2/article2 (accessed 1 February 2017).

McCormack, B. and Titchen, A. (2015) No beginning, no end: an ecology of human flourishing (extended version). Critical Creativity Blog, http://criticalcreativity.org/2014/08/19/no-beginning-no-end-an-ecology-of-human-flourishinan g-extended-version-2/(accessed 1 February 2017).

Peelo-Kilroe, L. (2014) Riding the heron: an experience of undertaking a creative visioning exercise with my critical creative companion, in second critical–creative retreat with Lorna – August 2014, Blog post. http://criticalcreativity.org/2014/08/13/circles-of-connection-a-critical-creative-companionship/(accessed 1 February 2017).

Polanyi, M. (1958) *Personal Knowledge: Towards a Post-Critical Philosophy*. University of Chicago Press, Chicago.

Polkinghorne, D.E. (1988) *Narrative Knowing and the Human Sciences*. State University of New York Press, Albany.

Ricoeur, P. (1976) *Interpretation Theory: Discourse and the Surplus of Meaning*. Texas Christian University Press, Fort Worth.

Rolfe, G. (2006) Validity, trustworthiness and rigour: quality and the idea of qualitative research. *Journal of Advanced Nursing*, **53**, 304–310.

Sælør, K.-T. and Biong, S. (2011) Endringer i sykepleieres arbeid etter rusreformen (Changes for nurses after the reform of health services for people living with substance abuse). *Sykepleien Forskning*, **6**, 170–176.

Titchen, A. (2015) Action research: genesis, evolution and orientations. *International Practice Development Journal*, **5**, Article 1. http://www.fons.org/library/journal/volume5-issue1/article1 (accessed 1 February 2017).

Titchen, A. and Ajjawi, R. (2010) Writing contemporary ontological and epistemological questions about practice, in *Researching Practice: A Discourse on Qualitative Methodologies* (eds J. Higgs, N. Cherry, R. Macklin and R. Ajjawi). Sense Publishers, Rotterdam. pp. 45–55.

Titchen, A. and Higgs, J. (2007) Exploring interpretive and critical philosophies, in *Being Critical and Creative in Qualitative Research* (eds J. Higgs, A. Titchen, D. Horsfall and H.B. Armstrong). Hampden Press, Sydney. pp. 56–68.

Titchen, A. and Hobson, D. (2015) Phenomenology, in *Research Methods in the Social Sciences* (eds B. Somekh and C. Lewin). Sage, London. pp. 121–130.

Titchen, A. and Horsfall, H. (2011a) Creative research landscapes and gardens: reviewing options and opportunities, in *Creative Spaces for Qualitative Researching: Living Research* (eds J. Higgs, A. Titchen, D. Horsfall and D. Bridges). Sense Publishers, Rotterdam. pp. 35–44.

Titchen, A. and Horsfall, D. (2011b) Embodying creative imagination and expression in qualitative research, in *Creative Spaces for Qualitative Researching: Living Research* (eds J. Higgs, A. Titchen, D. Horsfall and D. Bridges). Sense Publishers, Rotterdam. pp. 179–190.

Titchen, A. and McCormack, B. (2008) A methodological walk in the forest: critical creativity and human flourishing, in *International Practice Development in Nursing and Healthcare* (eds K. Manley, B. McCormack and V. Wilson). Blackwell, Oxford. pp. 59–83.

Titchen, A. and McCormack, B. (2010) Dancing with stones: critical creativity as methodology for human flourishing. *Educational Action Research: An International Journal*, **18**, 531–554.

4 Being a Person-Centred Researcher: Principles and Methods for Doing Research in a Person-Centred Way

Gaby Jacobs, Famke van Lieshout, Marit Borg and Ottar Ness

INTRODUCTION

Person-centredness has multiple origins, as described in Chapters 1 and 2 of this book. Some of the key origins are from humanistic–existential oriented models of care in the 1950–1960s (e.g. Hildegard Peplau and Carl Rogers) and 1970s (e.g. Joyce Travelbee), critical pedagogy from the 1970s onwards (e.g. Paulo Freire) and within the recovery-tradition in mental health from the 1980s (Borg, 2007; Davidson, Rakfeldt and Strauss, 2010). Person-centred approaches as professional practices and as a personal and political philosophy are often associated with the work of Carl Rogers (Rogers, 1961). The ultimate goal of a person-centred intervention is human growth and development, or in Rogers' terms 'becoming a person'. However, Rogers' work has been criticised for its individualistic and decontextualised approach. Other humanist approaches, like that of Freire (2007), have laid the ground for including relational empowerment and social justice as a core element in person-centred practice. Empowerment means that people become subjects of their own experience and actions as an essential part of full humanness. It is a relational and collective process that both promotes individual and group critical awareness, self-esteem and skills, as well as bringing about social and political change.

Following on from this positioning, we acknowledge that person-centredness and also person-centred research is an agenda for personal, collective and social transformation. Therefore, relational, contextual and political perspectives need to be included in research approaches and methods. A relational perspective is important since the interaction between persons, e.g. researchers and participants, is key in conducting research. Power relationships, different expectations, interests, needs, feelings and projections all make up the research relationship. Without making these explicit, they will be hidden and possibly hinder the processes and outcomes of research. Contextual perspectives are needed because the 'whole truth' needs to be attended to, including one's nationality, class, gender, ideology and sexuality, which make up a person's place and understanding in the world and influence the interaction. Political perspectives need to be considered, because doing person-centred research means challenging dominating ideologies and structures that prevent the 'becoming of a person' of human beings. This is often manifest in the

Person-Centred Healthcare Research, First Edition. Edited by Brendan McCormack, Sandra van Dulmen, Hilde Eide, Kirsti Skovdahl and Tom Eide.
© 2017 John Wiley & Sons Ltd. Published 2017 by John Wiley & Sons Ltd.

individualising or medicalising of human distress, thereby 'blaming the victim', instead of changing dysfunctional or unhealthy living and working environments (Proctor, 2006).

VALUES OF PERSON-CENTREDNESS

Previous chapters have provided an overview of the background of person-centredness and highlighted the potential value to draw on a wide range of person-centred values as the rudder for the formation of healthful relationships in research and practice – values such as respect, reciprocity, mutuality and self-determination (McCormack and McCance, 2010) impact upon a person's way of relating, including thinking, observing, listening and acting. In this chapter we consider these values as the foundation for principles of person-centredness in doing research and being a person-centred researcher. These show the relational character of person-centredness that should also underlie person-centred research. Furthermore, we support Proctor's (2006) emphasis on understanding person-centredness as an agenda for social change, meaning that contextual and political perspectives need to be included in research. Person-centredness so becomes a value-led and multi-layered approach to the way we conduct research.

PRINCIPLES OF PERSON-CENTRED RESEARCH

The key principle of person-centred research is derived from our relational and contextual view of person-centred practice and research. We have called this principle *connectivity*, which stands for the efforts to connect with oneself, other persons and contexts and which is expressed in the way one does research (doing), talks about it (knowing) and is as a researcher and person (being). This key principle gives direction for person-centred research in a research project. More specifically, it draws on two pairs of related principles, i.e. (i) attentiveness and dialogue, and (ii) empowerment and participation. These principles help the discussion on the roles, positions, methods, processes and outputs while doing research. Additionally, a third principle is needed to reflect on the way these principles are put into practice. This third principle is critical reflexivity regarding the process, context and outcomes of research.

The overall focus of this chapter is about how to make these principles 'work' in different phases of the research process. We illustrate the application of these principles in research, with a focus on action research, drawing on the many-faceted roots of person-centredness. Dilemmas and challenges will be addressed. Issues concerning research ethics will be reflected upon in relation to formal processes as well as human aspects.

We cannot be exhaustive in our presentation of methodologies and methods, because researchers may use many different approaches in accordance with their research questions, aims and objectives and the context in which they conduct their study. So by drawing on action research as an illustrative methodology, we hope to show that the person-centredness of doing research is not only set in specific methods, but also in the principles and stance that inform their application.

Main principle: Connectivity

Connectivity is inspired by the work of Gergen (2009) who states that people are in essence relational beings and that all meaning originates from coordinated action, including research action. Connectivity refers to the view that it is out of relationships that we as human beings grow and flourish and that knowledge, too, is co-constructed in the coaction of people; not linear and causal influence, but confluence as a relational view of agency is key in connectivity. Deleuze and Guattari (2004) introduced the idea of rhizomatics, outlining that our ways of thinking are like a rhizome, which acts like a complex and often non-logical underground matrix with no beginning or end, only 'in-betweens'. They also argued that we can get fixed in our thinking, so that we need to de-territorialise our position to become more nomadic in our thoughts and actions; opening up to other possibilities, perspectives and ways of being. Connectivity as a main principle of person-centred research puts forward the view that we do not do research *about* others, but do research *with* them as human beings. This is further outlined by three related principles.

Related principle 1: Attentiveness and dialogue

Attentiveness is a matter of seeing oneself, others, contexts and their interrelationship as human. It requires the capacity to be contextually aware, listen, and to see and to interpret sympathetically what we hear and what we see (Jordan, Walker and Hartling, 2004). This is a foundation of doing person-centred research. Attentiveness to the needs, values, viewpoints, aims and desires of the other person, to the relationship and to the context, is closely linked to the value of respect and to the therapeutic skills of empathy and compassion. In particular, in doing research with marginalised or in other ways vulnerable groups, attentiveness helps us to connect with the life situation, the choices and the sufferings of others, without becoming emotionally immersed in them or observing them dispassionately.

Dialogue is based on mutual attention and respect: recognising oneself and the other as a person that is worthwhile, which lends dignity and autonomy to the other and oneself (Bohm, 1996). Dialogue requires openness and transparency in relation to what or whom we attend to. When this succeeds, a social and communicative space is created in which experiences and knowledge are articulated, differences explored, shared meanings constructed and joint action taken (Bohm, 1996; Jacobs, 2010b). One of Bakhtin's (1984) main concerns was how to respectfully and creatively engage with others whose ideas and practices are different from one's own. Such a dialogic ideally welcomes and celebrates differences (Sampson, 1993), without forcing persons to speak and be understood within the familiarities and sensibilities of one discourse (i.e. the 'researchers').

Related principle 2: Empowerment and participation

Person-centred practice and research aim for the empowerment of individuals and groups by facilitating development into self-awareness and self-esteem, capacity building and (individual or collective) action. However, empowerment is a highly contested concept. Often empowerment is seen as respecting or fostering the autonomy of persons. The humanist notion of autonomy has been defined as independence, freedom from external control or influence, self-governance or self-steering. However, all of these conceptions ignore the interdependence of human beings, as feminist theorists like Jessica Benjamin (cf. Benjamin, 2010) and Judith Butler (cf. Butler, 2015) have argued. They have put forward the notion of relational autonomy, in which human beings are seen as intersubjectively constituted and socially embedded, and at the same time capable of self-determination or moral and political agency, i.e. making choices regarding one's own life project. Empowerment then is a relational and multilevel (intrapersonal, interpersonal, organisational and societal) construct that refers to human development within relationships and contexts. In person-centred research we need to acknowledge that many groups we do research with, feel marginalised and powerless. Empowerment then means that they gain mastery over their lives (Deegan, 1997).

Participation is critical in this process, as well as an outcome in itself. Participation is having a voice in choices and actions that matter, working in partnership or organising oneself with the support of others. It allows for different sorts and degrees of participation and can contribute to empowerment with the right level of challenge and support (Jacobs, 2010a). Participation always takes place within a context of power relationships, that may have three different faces (Jacobs, 2001; Tew, 2006): *power over*, i.e. hierarchical relationships in which one dominates over the other; *power with*, i.e. the sharing of strengths and resources in order to become stronger collectively; and *power to*, i.e. the transformative power of different stakeholders working together and struggling to act for a better world (or practice). Only the latter two can be part of a person-centred approach of doing research, since these contribute to human flourishing and wellbeing whereas domination does not.

Related principle 3: Critical reflexivity

Within research, critical reflexivity is needed to understand what power relationships are fostered and maintained and who benefits from them. Power relationships in society related to gender, ethnicity, social class, age and the like, also confluence with the research setting and relationships. Concerns about the unexamined power of the researcher led to a focus on reflexivity that aimed to reframe power balances between participants and researchers (Finlay and Gough, 2003). Hertz (1997), for instance, urges researchers to be aware of their own positions and interests and to explicitly situate themselves within the research. She argues that:

> researchers are...imposed at all stages of the research process – from the questions they ask to those they ignore, from who they study to who they ignore, from problem formulation to analysis, representation and writing – in order to produce less distorted accounts of the social world. (p. viii)

Finlay and Gough (2003) emphasise that the reflexive researcher looks through a critical lens at the process, context and outcomes of research and interrogates the construction of knowledge. In order for dialogue as the co-construction of meaning to be able to happen, participants have to reflect on the conditions under which the dialogue (or broader: the research project) is taking place, the assumptions underpinning it and the power relationships that lead to inclusion and exclusion of persons, perspectives and actions (Bohm, 1996; Burbules, 2000).

THE APPLICATION OF PERSON-CENTRED PRINCIPLES IN RESEARCH: A CASE EXAMPLE

Applying these person-centred principles in research means:

1. having a strong focus on the relationships with others (caregivers and caretakers/service users, co-researchers, etc.), as well as on power issues in the research process with an overall intent to knowledge co-construction, as well as individual, team and contextual growth as a person-centred outcome;

2. striving for an appropriate level and nature of participation for ourselves as researchers, service users, practitioners, lay people and/or family members in all phases of the research process: establishing the research group, the choice for and ways of applying methods of data collections and analysis, and in disseminating results;

3. striving for the research to be systematic and rigorous as well as to take deliberate action to meet the quality criteria congruent to the principles of person-centredness. Such a relational and contextual stance shapes the research findings and products ('knowing') and the 'doing' by the researchers in context;

4. a person-centred stance is part of, and also shapes the 'being' of the researcher, which is in a constant interplay with the 'doing' and 'knowing' and therefore fosters professional and personal growth (van Lieshout, 2013). Reflexivity regarding our relational being as researchers and its development is therefore also a key characteristic of person-centred research.

In this part of the chapter we will demonstrate what it entails to try to apply these person-centred principles within research, by referring to several research projects published in the literature.

Case 1: A collaborative mental health project

The research context is an action research project in a Municipality in Southeast Norway – a collaboration between the Centre for Mental Health and Substance Abuse (we will call it the Centre from here) at The University College of Southeast Norway, the municipality (a local government district), the local service user and family member organisations.

Our aim was to focus our research on issues emerging through discussions with practice practitioners, service users and family members in clinical settings (Ness *et al.*, 2014). This concrete project started through a meeting between representatives from the Centre and practitioners in various roles working in mental health and substance abuse settings. The meeting was initiated by the Centre and its purpose was to see if there could be any interest in research collaboration based on the needs of the municipality. There was a positive interest in research collaboration. The municipality underlined their limited experience and time to be involved in the proposal work; therefore the Centre took responsibility for the proposal-work for a funding application to the National Research Council of Norway. Following a number of discussions, it was agreed that the research focus would relate to services for young people experiencing co-occurring mental health and substance use problems. The more concrete questions the municipality was interested in were:

1. How do service users, family members and practitioners experience services and collaboration in these service contexts?

2. Is it possible to develop a composite model for collaboration and coordination in mental health and substance abuse services drawing on these lived experiences?

We were also interested in the possible transferability of such a model developed in a concrete setting to other parts of the municipality as well as the country.

Reflecting on this first phase, we would do things differently now. At the start of the project development, we didn't have contacts with local service user/family members in the municipality, so these partners did not participate from the beginning. However, this is rather typical of the starting phase of a research project where a research centre plays a major part in the project development and where the format of the research application has an impact on the process, as we will also see in the other case.

After getting the research funding from the National Research Council, the Centre initiated a meeting where all partners were present. This involved researchers, leaders and practitioners from the municipality and people from service user and family member organisations meeting to design and plan the research. The first action was to decide collaboratively on the scope of the project, which happened in several dialogue meetings. These dialogue meetings included young adults (aged 18–28) with co-occurring mental health and substance use problems (people with lived experience), family members and practitioners. As well as clarifying the project scope, the time spent together also helped to develop shared understandings and descriptions of collaboration. A steering group of leaders from the research project, the University College, the municipality and the service user and family member organisations was established.

As a part of the action research methodology, we had two strategies for involving people with lived experience. First, we recruited a sociologist with lived experience to a 50% position in the project in order to strengthen the position of experience-based research and knowledge. In this, 'attentiveness and dialogue' was a key principle being employed. Secondly, we established a 'competence group' to work in close participation with the research team in all stages of the study. The competence group consisted of two family members, two service users, and three practitioners from the municipality. Inspired by the concept of participatory research this competence group of 'co-researchers' participated in developing the research project in detail, e.g. working out the interview guides and inclusion criteria, advising on the interview situations, data analysis, and in the ongoing planning and discussions of the entire study. The competence group met four times annually throughout the project. Researchers and co-researchers worked collaboratively in identifying problems, deciding on themes for inquiry, selecting a research design, and designing projects for implementation. Data were collected by multistaged focus group interviews (practitioners and family members), and in-depth qualitative interviews (young adults). The researcher with lived experience performed all interviews along with another researcher, and they also jointly conducted the analysis and the writing of papers for publication.

In the last phase of the project we collaborated with the municipality and other associated organisations to determine how the preliminary findings could be made use of in daily situations. We met with practitioners and talked with them about the findings from our research. Then we discussed together with them how they could use the findings as part of their work. We held evening meetings with service users and family members in order to discuss how they would see the findings being used by the municipality. A one-day seminar was held to present all the findings in the research project.

Making research an ethical and collaborative effort has empowered the different stakeholders (service users, family members and practitioners) in using research outcomes while the research is ongoing. This involves acknowledging the good work people are already doing, as well as making important changes in the services and use of collaborative practice in mental health and substance abuse care.

Case 2: Participatory action research for healthy living

The second case was a Participatory Action Research (PAR) project with older persons from a Moroccan and Dutch background in the Netherlands, focusing on 'healthy living' (Jacobs, 2010a). This methodology was chosen because of its contribution to empowerment of the communities of older people, which was one of the project goals. The other goal was the development of an intervention programme for promoting healthy living amongst older people in the Netherlands and contributing to the knowledge base on healthy living. The project team consisted of a heterogeneous group of people: eight older people (50+) living in Rotterdam with a low socio-economic status – four of them were born in the Netherlands and four of them emigrated from Morocco between 20 and 30 years earlier. They were the key persons to help include the wider community's voices in the project by conducting interviews and feeding back the results. Working with the community members were two health practitioners (one from the municipal health agency, the other from a national health agency specialising in the development of multicultural health practices), three researchers from the university and the project manager (a university professor). All project members were paid for their contribution, including the participants from the community, in order to establish an equal partnership with the older people as co-researchers, co-developers and co-educators.

In the first stage of the project the researchers and health agencies were looking for funding and wrote up the project proposal. Community members were not participating in this stage, because of the high time pressure to get the proposal in, but the proposal only stated a general goal in order to have space to fill in the details with input from the community members them-selves. Once the grant was received, we formed the project group as outlined previously. In the first 6 months of the project, the group met monthly to discuss the goals of the project and to design the data collection phase. However, after this first stage, time pressure increased and in order to work more efficiently, the project group was split into a research group, a practice group and a community group. The participation level of community members in the research dropped as did the involvement of researchers in the health agency's practice and in the communities. This continued until the end of the project, resulting in dissatisfaction and feelings of disempowerment for most participants. The relational dynamics within this project were analysed by using the theory of organisational learning and especially the notion of 'defensive routines' developed by Argyris and Schön (1978). This provided insights into the difficulties experienced in keeping dialogue, reflection and learning going within a context of external pressure and also to learn from this experience for future projects. However, most significantly we learned about the challenges associated with realising the principle of 'empowerment and participation' in research.

Case 3: The dialogue project – a narrative study

This case highlights the central place of 'critical reflexivity' in research. From 2010 to 2013 we were involved in the research group 'Professional Values in Critical Dialogue' from Fontys University of Applied Sciences (Jacobs, 2010b). This group started a qualitative study into the Master Course Special Educational Needs (M SEN) for teachers working within the field of education (Jacobs, 2013). We wanted to know what contribution the Master Course made to the professional development of these teachers.

In the first stage of the project, we organised four dialogue group meetings; two meetings with lecturers and two meetings with course coordinators (24 participants in total). The goal of these meetings was to bring into dialogue the ideals of educators within the M SEN course regarding the professional development of teachers. The two main research questions were:

1. *What* do educators in the M SEN aim for in the course or the parts they teach?
2. *How* do they (try to) achieve this?

First we asked the participants to think about these questions and to write down their response on a sheet of paper by completing two sentences:

1. What I want to achieve with my students is…
2. I do this by….

After this moment of individual reflection, we started the dialogue, by asking the participants to bring in their responses on paper to these questions. At the end of the session, we asked the participants to tell us whether during the dialogue anything else came to their mind that they considered important regarding the topic of this meeting.

We facilitated the dialogue as researchers. The task of the facilitators was to encourage dialogical narrative interventions. At the same time, we took part in the dialogue ourselves, by bringing in experiences and knowledge we had from the course and our own teaching; and to provoke diversity when agreement seemed to dominate and vice versa.

The dialogue meetings were taped on a digital voice recorder and fully transcribed. A narrative thematic analysis was conducted by reconstructing storylines and troubles in the dialogues (Kohler Riessman, 2008). Storylines refer to the recurring themes throughout the dialogue, and the co-construction of meanings around these themes. Our main interest was in the higher goals the lecturers attributed to the course, and the means to achieve these goals. Troubles refer to the tensions between these goals and means, or between different meanings given to similar goals or means. Troubles also include barriers or the lack of necessary conditions to achieve the intended goals or employ the desirable means. The narrative analysis was first conducted separately by the two researchers and then brought into a critical dialogue to enhance our reflexivity in the research project. We also spent a research group meeting on a panel analysis of the material, in which the thematic framework was further developed.

In our project we built in a method to see whether the dialogue would contribute to the critical reflection of the participants by asking the participants to fill in a short questionnaire twice, once at the beginning and the second time at the end of the dialogue group meeting. Comparing their answers to these two questionnaires showed that the dialogue meetings themselves made participants aware of tacit views and meanings, thereby contributing to their professional development as teachers and as human beings. By hearing others' viewpoints and confronting them with their own, their own views became stronger, broadened or transformed.

Participants were asked to write down their reflections on the dialogue group meeting and to send them by email to the researchers. These emails showed that the dialogue meetings also triggered the motivation for action of some participants; they not only wanted to discuss pedagogical issues with colleagues but also wanted to start small action research projects within their own teaching practice. Therefore, the dialogue meetings not only were useful as a data collection method, but also as a developmental tool within the department and curriculum. As a research method, they helped to co-construct tacit pedagogical views (values), goals and means, and to discover the tensions between them. As an intervention method, the dialogical process triggered a learning and a questioning attitude amongst (in this case) educators, resulting in enthusiasm and energy with educators to develop small (action) research projects within the curriculum. Most importantly, participants felt empowered by speaking together about their teaching practice and underlying values with colleagues. The sharing of stories in a setting that was characterised by attention and positive regard, as well as their participation in the analysis of their dialogues, contributed to feelings of relational agency: being part of a shared endeavour to further improve higher education practice.

CONCLUSION

The case examples show the strengths and possibilities as well as the difficulties of applying person-centred principles in research practice. Especially when underlying values or interests and goals clash, which is often the case in collaborative research, relational processes may become degenerative instead of generative (Jordan, Walker and Hartling, 2004; Gergen, 2009). The participation of community members to a high degree in all project stages should not be seen as the golden rule; rather as an aim to strive for when the internal and external conditions are often not optimal, which is often the case. Whatever research methodology or method is chosen, attentiveness and dialogue, participation and empowerment, as well as critical reflexivity are key in practising person-centred research. These principles contribute to connectivity: the coaction of participants and confluence of happenings that lead to transformation, on a personal, collective and social/political level. There is no recipe for doing person-centred research and no easy way out of relational challenges, but as Walker (2001) reminds us:

> The purpose is to work optimistically with the possible, for all its limits, rather than only pessimistically reiterating the hopeless. (p. 31)

REFERENCES

Argyris, C. and Schon, D. (1978) *Organizational Learning: A Theory of Action Perspective.* Addison Wesley, Reading.

Bahktin, M. (2004) Dialogic origin and dialogic pedagogy of grammar: stylistics in teaching Russian language in secondary school. Trans. Lydia Razran Stone. *Journal of Russian and East European Psychology,* **42**, 12–49.

Benjamin, J. (2010) Where's the gap and what's the difference?: the relational view of intersubjectivity, multiple selves and enactments. *Contemporary Psychoanalysis,* **46**, 112–119.

Bohm, D. (1996) *On Dialogue.* Routledge, New York.

Borg, M. (2007) *The Nature of Recovery as Lived in Everyday Life: Perspectives of Individuals Recovering from Severe Mental Health Problems.* PhD dissertation. Institute of Social Work and Health Sciences, NTNU, Trondheim, Norway.

Burbules, N.C. (2000) The limits of dialogue as a critical pedagogy, in *Revolutionary Pedagogies* (ed. P.P. Trifonas). Routledge, New York. pp. 251–272.

Butler, J. (2015) *Senses of the Subject.* Fordham University Press, New York.

Davidson, L., Rakfeldt, J. and Strauss, J. (2010) *The Roots of the Recovery Movement in Psychiatry.* Wiley Blackwell, Oxford.

Deegan, P.E. (1997) Recovery and empowerment for people with psychiatric disabilities. *Social Work in Health Care,* **25**, 11–24.

Deleuze, G. and Guattari, F. (2004) *A Thousand Plateaus.* Continuum, London.

Finlay, L. and Gough, B. (eds) (2003) *Reflexivity: A Practical Guide for Researchers in Health and Social Science.* Blackwell Publishing, Oxford.

Freire, P. (2007) *Pedagogy of the Oppressed.* Continuum, New York.

Gergen, K. (2009) *Relational Being. Beyond Self and Community.* Oxford University Press, Oxford.

Hertz, R. (ed.) (1997) *Reflexivity and Voice.* Sage, London.

Jacobs, G. (2013) Conflicting views on professional development. Critical dialogue as a research and intervention method for a master's course in professional education for teachers. *Journal of Social Intervention: Theory and Practice,* **22**, 4–22.

Jacobs, G. (2001) *De paradox van kracht en kwetsbaarheid. Empowerment in feministisch hulpverlening en humanistisch raadswerk.* SWP, Amsterdam. [The paradox of power and vulnerability. Empowerment in feminist and humanist counselling. Dissertation.]

Jacobs, G. (2010a) Conflicting demands and the power of defensive routines in participatory action research. *Action Research,* **8**, 367–386.

Jacobs, G. (2010b) *Professional Values in Critical Dialogue. Dealing with Uncertainty in Educational Practice*. Fontys University of Applied Sciences, Eindhoven.

Jordan, J., Walker, M. and Hartling L.M. (2004) *The Complexity of Connection*. Writings from the Stone Center, Boston.

Kohler Riessman, C. (2008) *Narrative Methods for the Human Sciences*. Sage, London.

Lieshout van, F. (2013) *Taking Action for Action. A Study of the Interplay between Contextual and Facilitator Characteristics in Developing an Effective Workplace Culture in a Dutch Hospital Setting, Through Action Research*. PhD Thesis, University of Ulster, Belfast.

Ness, O., Borg, M., Semb, R. and Karlsson, B. (2014) 'Walking alongside': collaborative practices in mental health and substance use care. *International Journal of Mental Health Systems*, **8**, 55.

McCormack, B. and McCance, T. (2010) *Person-Centred Nursing; Theory, Models and Methods*. Wiley Blackwell, Oxford.

Proctor, G. (2006) Therapy: opium of the masses or help for those who least need it?, in *Politicizing the Person-Centred Approach: An Agenda for Social Change* (eds G. Proctor, M. Cooper, P. Sanders and B. Malcolm). PCCS Books Ltd, Ross-on-Wye. pp. 66–79.

Rogers, C. (1961) *On Becoming a Person: A Therapist's View of Psychotherapy*. Constable, London.

Sampson, E. (1993) *Celebrating the Other: A Dialogic Account of Human Nature*. Westview Press, San Fransisco.

Tew, J. (2006) Understanding power and powerlessness. towards a framework for emancipatory practice in social work. *Journal of Social Work*, **6**, 33–51.

Walker, M. (ed.) (2001) *Reconstructing Professionalism in University Teaching. Teachers and Learners in Action*. SRHE/Open University Press, Buckingham.

5 Research into Person-Centred Healthcare Technology: A Plea for Considering Humanisation Dimensions

Gaby Jacobs, Teatske van der Zijpp, Famke van Lieshout and Sandra van Dulmen

INTRODUCTION

Changes in demographics, financial and time constraints and the on-going shift towards greater responsibility for health and illness for the patient, have increased the speed of development of innovative, information and communications technology-guided solutions and tools within healthcare practices. Telecare technologies, e-health and smart home developments provide practical solutions for the 'problems' of the ageing population, such as the increasing levels of chronic illness and the rising demand for health and social care, as well as the shortage of staff and financial strains on health and welfare budgets (Roberts and Mort, 2009). Technology facilitates communication through email, websites, electronic monitors and webcams to interact with patients, to monitor them, to transmit data and to provide instructions. The hands-on care of the healthcare provider can be replaced or supplemented by technology: an 'app', a 'tablet', a website, a computer, or even a robot. Technology has thus become an inextricable part of today's healthcare practices. Although these developments are primarily driven by the aim to make healthcare more efficient and effective, they also trigger new and interesting research questions from a person-centred perspective.

TECHNOLOGY AND HUMANISATION

Person-centredness is a humanising principle in healthcare and other practices, aimed at high-quality relationships that are growth-fostering and empowering to all those involved (Jacobs, 2015). Doing person-centred research into technology in healthcare shifts the perspective from 'what is' and 'what is possible' (in technology) to 'what is desirable' from a perspective of humanisation. Humanisation literally means: to make human. It can be generally defined as cultivating working and living cultures within equitable institutions and, in a sustainable world, society that contributes to people's sense of meaning, strength and belonging (Nussbaum, 2006). A healthcare practice can manifest itself in eight dimensions that constitute a continuum from humanisation to dehumanisation (Todres, Galvin and Holloway,

Person-Centred Healthcare Research, First Edition. Edited by Brendan McCormack, Sandra van Dulmen, Hilde Eide, Kirsti Skovdahl and Tom Eide.
© 2017 John Wiley & Sons Ltd. Published 2017 by John Wiley & Sons Ltd.

2009). The extent to which a healthcare practice is humanising is determined by each of these eight dimensions (see Table 5.1). For example, installing all kinds of medical equipment for a person with chronic obstructive pulmonary disease can help that person to monitor his own health. However, as health includes more than physical functioning, there is a risk when a person is constantly reminded of his or her illness (reductionist body).

These humanisation dimensions could serve to secure the level of person-centredness in healthcare technology research. For the sake of this chapter, we have clustered the eight aspects into three broader themes that illustrate person-centredness:

1. Empowerment (including the dimensions of insiderness, agency and personal journey);
2. Relationship (including togetherness, sense of place);
3. Autonomy/dignity (including uniqueness, sense-making and embodiment).

We discuss these themes through studies that use a, more or less, implicit, humanistic perspective. Therefore, we searched the literature for implications of using technology in care for person-centred practice with a special focus on ethics, relationships and empowerment (see Box 5.1). In the next sections, we explore how care relationships change when introducing technology. Secondly, we analyse the contribution of technology to empowerment and recognition of agency of care consumers and caregivers. Lastly, we discuss the implications of technology for autonomy and dignity of persons in healthcare. Finally, we will conclude with a reflection on what we have learned about person-centred research into technology in healthcare, by looking at the different studies into these topics.

Table 5.1 Conceptual framework of the dimensions of humanisation.

Forms of humanisation	Forms of dehumanisation
Insiderness	Objectification
Agency	Passivity
Uniqueness	Homogenisation
Togetherness	Isolation
Sense-making	Loss of meaning
Personal journey	Loss of personal journey
Sense of place	Dislocation
Embodiment	Reductionist body

Source: Courtesy of Todres, Galvin and Halloway (2009, p. 70).

Box 5.1   Literature review

A database search was conducted using the databases CINAHL and PubMed. These databases were utilised because of their focus on health and nursing. Search terms included 'person-centred*' or 'person centered', 'ethic*', 'relation*', 'empowerment' combined with 'technol*'. An advanced search strategy was used with the restriction that the search terms were present in the abstract and published between 2010 and 2015. In addition, a manual search was done on the reference lists. This resulted in 19 studies being included in the review.

TECHNOLOGY AND THE HEALTHCARE RELATIONSHIP

Several studies have been conducted into the impact of the use of technology on the health-care relationship. What happens for example if direct care is replaced or supplemented by telecare? The potential consequence of being monitored and cared for from a distance 24 hours a day, is that face-to-face contact and hands-on care diminish. Research has shown that caregivers fear that care will become a poor version of what they value and aim at, i.e. the core values and goals of professional work (May *et al.*, 2001; Roberts and Mort, 2009; Mort *et al.*, 2015). Mort *et al.* (2015) argue that technology offers no 'technological fix' to replace either existing healthcare services or informal care networks. Roberts and Mort (2009) on the other hand pose that telecare only deals with monitoring tasks and leaves the physical care and social emotional care untouched. Others express ethical concerns around realising values and beliefs such as compassion in contributing to the wellbeing of their care recipients and bonding with team members (Nieboer *et al.*, 2014). This fear is supported by research that shows that care and attention cannot be replaced by technology, because technology has no emotions and cannot deal with unexpected interactions (Sparrow and Sparrow, 2006). Critics have argued that this is the dehumanising force of technology: the 'heart' is taken out of care. However, in practice-oriented research, no evidence is found for the distinction between 'cold and distant technologies' versus 'warm and close care'.

In a study by Pols (2012) nurses expressed the fear that telecare practices would hinder the development of good relations with service users. A telecommunication modem was installed in the person's home (a small white box) that would ask them every morning the same questions about their physical, social and emotional health. Whenever the person gave an answer that required action, a nurse would ring in to have a chat and give instructions. The study showed that service users experienced this device as a warm and caring technology. It not only strengthened their relationships with caregivers, but also with relatives, because the questions also helped them to talk to their family members about their condition. The technology therefore was supporting relationships, rather than disrupting or replacing them (Pols, 2012). Moreover, a systematic review by Morris *et al.* (2014) suggests that the use of technology can improve social connectivity and the degree to which a person experiences togetherness through contact with others. They selected 14 studies that showed positive results of smart technology on social support. However, mixed results were found for empowerment as well as for measures of loneliness. When looking at the six studies that included face-to-face contacts next to technology, five out of these six studies demonstrated positive findings for measures of social connectivity and quality of life. This review study shows emerging evidence that technology can improve some dimensions of social connectedness such as social support and self-efficacy. However, it also suggests that more research is needed into the benefits of face-to-face contact in addition to smart technologies.

Clearly, technological devices change the relationships in care practices and the relationships in the social world. These changes create opportunities for new and meaningful connections between caregivers and care receivers and between peers, but they also raise moral questions and risks. A view in which technology is 'external' or 'instrumental' to care relationships does not do justice to technology as meaningful within the interaction between persons (Jordal, Heggen and Nyheim Solbrække, 2015). From a person-centred perspective, therefore, we need to ask how technology influences relationships – the social connectedness of human beings – and how it contributes to humanistic values or diminishes them.

EMPOWERMENT OF USERS AND RECOGNITION OF PERSONHOOD

Empowerment is a multidimensional process in which individuals, groups and communities acquire self-esteem, critical consciousness, and the skills to determine their own lives, health and environment (Zimmerman, 1995). Characteristic of an empowerment approach in healthcare is the focus on possibilities and resilience instead of problems and dysfunction. It fits with a positive and proactive notion of health (Huber *et al.*, 2011) and is a key outcome of person-centred practice (McCormack and McCance, 2010).

Healthcare technology has the potential to contribute to the self-management or empowerment of service users, especially for people with chronic diseases living in remote areas or for people with difficulty accessing care. It enables them to become actively involved in their disease management process and access information related to their condition, which increases their agency and control over their own lives and health. For care providers it offers possibilities for remote data interpretation and the provision of timely interventions (Demiris, Doorenbos and Towle, 2009; Suter, Suter and Johnston, 2011). However, research shows that this promise of empowerment of service-users and the promotion of disease management are not easily achieved and that technology may reinforce dependency, passivity and control by caregivers instead of improving self-management, which is dehumanising instead of humanising (Todres, Galvin and Holloway, 2009). In a telecare project for persons with heart failure it was found that a monitoring device for measuring vital signs daily at home shifted responsibility 'for spotting trouble from the patient to the nurse' (Pols, 2012, p.67). However, at the same time the values of good care shifted towards prevention by early intervention and away from values of self-help, cautious medical intervention and service user initiative. As a consequence of the monitoring device, 'patients felt safe (rather than responsible) and well looked after by their nurses' (Pols, 2012, p.59). This issue of safety will be elaborated upon in the next section.

From a person-centred perspective we might ask if these service users were empowered by using the device? Did it increase taking account of insiderness (i.e. their subjectivity), agency and personal journey? Schermer (2014) argues that in many cases the service user remains dependent on professionals because it is the caregiver who interprets the data and decides if and what action should be taken. This means that professionals manage the person and his or her disease from a distance based on 'how' the person is and not so much on 'who' the person is, which implies a loss of personal journey (Todres, Galvin and Holloway, 2009). The service user only has a supporting and executing role and learns to live the prescribed lifestyle. Moreover, Schermer (2014) argues that self-management requires that care receivers are able to recognise symptoms and can act adequately, that they are able and willing to fit the lifestyle recommendations into their own lifestyle and that they can handle the physical and psychosocial impact of their disease. However, in reality persons make choices that are not in agreement with evidence-based guidelines but do fit in with their personal history and future aspirations. These choices are based on their own values, beliefs and preferences, which are experienced as meaningful, but can be in conflict with professional guidelines and norms. Also, self-management is often not experienced as an empowering concept by persons themselves (Bagchus and Dedding, 2015), because it individualises problems and does not acknowledge the person's personal journey, including their vulnerability as well as their strengths. It is perceived that to manage oneself, i.e. to take care of oneself, one needs to be in good health. For persons with a chronic disease, this is not the case. They express the need to be cared for and to be eased from the responsibility to manage their care (and the different caregivers), and the longing for someone who is present and compassionate.

From a person-centred perspective it is therefore important to acknowledge how caregivers and care consumers perceive suitable care. According to Pols (2012, p. 45) 'it may aim for patient independence in some situations, whereas it would mean close professional monitoring in others'. Technology in healthcare does not create new dilemmas when it comes to empowerment, but it forces us to revisit the old ones, such as the tension between 'taking control' and 'leaning back' in order for the person to use one's voice and capacities for self-determination (Jacobs, 2010). We have to ask ourselves as caregivers and researchers: what is needed here, for whom and for what? And how do we know?

AUTONOMY, DIGNITY AND SAFETY

A third theme of humanisation involves the contribution of healthcare practices to a person's autonomy, dignity and safety. Research shows that dilemmas arise when using technology, because it can interfere with these values (Zwijsen, Niemeijer and Hertogh, 2011; Landau and Werner, 2012; Niemeijer *et al.*, 2015). This can be illustrated by the example of surveillance technology (assistive technology). This concerns devices such as electronic bracelets, global positioning systems (GPS), video and audio surveillance, and movement sensors.

On the one hand, the use of assistive technology is considered to enhance personal freedom and consequently autonomy, for instance for persons with dementia. On the other hand, this technology is found to impact on individuals' privacy and dignity. For example, in an ethnographic field study using observations and interviews by Niemeijer *et al.* (2015), it was found that some persons did benefit from surveillance technology, for example as a means of engaging with new spaces. However, others felt stigmatised, missed the company of support workers or did not want to 'be watched'. According to Niemeijer (2015, p. 318) 'surveillance technology in residential care should not be approached in a black and white manner, as being either positive or negative, but rather as something which can only contribute to the autonomy of clients if it is set in a truly person-centred approach, tailored to the individual with his strength and needs'.

This links to the dimension of 'uniqueness' in the framework of humanisation developed by Todres, Galvin and Holloway (2009). They warrant for the tendency in practice that 'in order to "fit in", one may adopt the role of a "good patient" acting according to expectation, not complaining and complying with treatment' (Todres, Galvin and Holloway, 2009, p. 71). However, while being sick, people want to maintain dignity by 'maintaining the self' and retaining personal identity as a unique individual. Another dilemma that is discussed in the literature concerns the tension between values of autonomy on the one hand and safety on the other. According to Landau and Werner (2012) it is often not the maximisation of autonomy but rather safety (the drive for protecting the person from harm) that was considered as the decisive argument of caregivers to use surveillance technology. However, at the same time, safety causes tension with autonomy. For example, to guarantee optimal safety (and no false sense of security), in monitoring persons by using sensors, these sensors should be installed in all rooms of a personal living environment. Without an alert to a person who is ready to act on the other side of the monitoring device, no safety can be promised. However, being watched constantly by monitoring devices could cause serious feelings of violation of privacy (Zwijsen, Niemeijer and Hertogh, 2011). This focus on safety instead of autonomy can be seen as an example of a 'reductionist view of the body' (to protect it from harm) and a neglect of a more relational view of the body in its broader meaningful context such as psychological, environmental, social and spiritual matrices conflicting with the dimension of embodiment (Todres, Galvin and Holloway, 2009).

To conclude, it is important to acknowledge that the use of technological innovations creates potential tension for person-centred values such as autonomy, dignity and safety. While the technology claims to increase autonomy, there is the risk that this infringes on dignity or safety.

CHARACTERISTICS OF PERSON-CENTRED RESEARCH INTO TECHNOLOGY IN HEALTHCARE PRACTICES

When looking at the literature on technology in healthcare from a person-centred perspective, we posed the following questions:

1. What does research into the humanising or dehumanising consequences of technology in healthcare practices teach us?
2. What are the characteristics of this kind of research and what insights are still lacking?

We identified three key themes.

Broadened research questions

What we found is that research into the humanising consequences of technology in healthcare practices is different from other technology studies in that it does not (only) ask questions about the effectiveness or efficiency of technologies. It is interested in the ethics of technology, the attitudes towards technology of different stakeholders, user involvement in development, implementation and decision-making, and the implications on relationships in healthcare and beyond. The focus on relationships seems central to research from a person-centred perspective. It means that these studies don't just focus on the evaluation of technologies, but they also focus on the evaluation of the relationships that people and technologies create. This also sheds a different light on studies that look at the implications for autonomy and independence. A view of persons as social and reciprocal beings, which is central to person-centredness, does not propose to foster coping skills, self-management, independent living or social connectedness only through technological means unless this is the personal journey a person prefers. This also implies that in initiating and developing technology-supported healthcare interventions, the service user's voice should count most. Ideally, in every step of the development process, service users' needs, preferences, perspectives and experiences should be actively sought and taken into account (van Bruinessen *et al.*, 2014). Such a user-centred approach is not only recommended by virtue of being person-centred and humane, but also increases the chance that service users as well as health providers accept, use and implement the resulting technology-supported intervention in daily life and/or healthcare.

Mixed methodologies

To receive insight into the central question as to how relationships change in and through technologies, participant observation and interviews, as well as focus groups are used. Quantitative studies alone will not reveal subtle changes in relationships, empowerment, dignity, autonomy and/or safety from a person-centred perspective. The closer the researcher gets to the practice studied (insider and user-perspective), the more insight is given into the complexity and dynamics within practice. The use of technology leads to mixed outcomes depending on the persons involved and their values, beliefs and preferences, the healthcare context and the kind of technology used. What fits and is perceived as humanising cannot be determined beforehand. Qualitative research, especially creative- and arts-based approaches, does throw light on this complexity and the ethical ambivalence and dilemmas involved. Additionally, creative- and arts-based approaches can be used to reveal emotional, affective and unconscious aspects (Coats, 2001; Argyris, 2010). By uncovering tacit knowledge that would otherwise remain hidden, and revealing ways of being that would otherwise remain unexamined, the opportunities for action can be increased (Higgs and Titchen, 2007; Simons and McCormack, 2007). It thereby helps to develop ethical frameworks that provide guidelines in using technology within healthcare practices (e.g. Mort *et al.*, 2015).

Future questions

As the literature review showed, technology changes the relationships in care practices thereby contributing to or hindering the practice of humanistic values, such as empowerment, autonomy, dignity and safety as outlined in the framework by Todres, Galvin and Holloway (2009). Several tensions were found, between autonomy and safety or dignity, and also between empowerment and control. From a person-centred perspective, we need to include the views of all persons when deciding if and how technology is used. However, this may be part of the problem, because the autonomy of the service user could conflict with safety from a healthcare perspective. More research is needed to entangle this and other moral dilemmas produced by technology from a person-centred perspective. Also research into other humanistic values is needed. So far, we haven't found studies that look at the impact of technology on a person's sense of place, which is also a dimension of relationship and thereby of humanisation.

CONCLUSION

Technology-supported healthcare can be humanising and dehumanising at the same time. When applying technology, it is important to consider and secure different aspects of person-centredness and regularly monitor end users' needs, experiences and perspectives. Mixed methodologies contribute to enhanced person-centred use of technologies in healthcare and throw light on promoting factors as well as obstacles to implementation, and the dilemmas that are part of this.

REFERENCES

Argyris, C. (2010) *Organisational Traps: Leadership, Culture, Organisational Design.* Oxford University Press, Oxford.

Bagchus, C. and Dedding, C. (2015) *Zelfmanagement. De kloof tussen beleidstaal en de ervaringen van ouderen met kanker.* Athena Instituut, VU, Amsterdam.

Bruinessen, I.R. van, Weel-Baumgarten, E.M. van, Snippe, H.W. *et al.* (2014) User driven eHealth. Patient participatory development and testing of a computer tailored communication training for patients with malignant lymphoma. *JMIR Research Protocols*, **3**, e59.

Coats, E. (2001) Weaving the body, the creative unconscious, imagination and the arts into practice development, in *Professional Practice in Health, Education and the Creative Arts* (eds J. Higgs and A. Titchen). Blackwell Science, Oxford. pp. 251–263.

Demiris, G., Doorenbos, A.Z. and Towle, C. (2009) Ethical considerations regarding the use of technology for older adults: the case of telehealth. *Research in Gerontological Nursing*, **2**, 128–136.

Higgs, J. and Titchen, A. (2007) Qualitative research: journeys of meaning making through transformation, illumination, shared action and liberation, in *Being Critical and Creative in Qualitative Research* (eds J. Higgs, A. Titchen, D. Horsfall and H. Armstrong). Hampden Press, Sydney. pp. 11–21.

Huber, M., Green, L., van der Horst, H., *et al.* (2011) How should we define Health? *BMJ*, **343**, d4163.

Jacobs, G. (2011) 'Take control or lean back?': barriers to practicing empowerment in health promotion. *Health Promotion Practice*, **12**, 94–101.

Jacobs, G. (2015) *Ont-wikkelen van verbindingen. Persoonsgerichte en evidence based praktijkvoering in zorg en welzijn*. Lectorale rede. Fontys Hogeschool Mens en Gezondheid, Eindhoven.

Jordal, K., Heggen, K. and Solbrække, K.N. (2015) Exploring the relationship between technology and care: a qualitative study of clinical practice for nursing students. *Journal of Nursing Education and Practice*, **5**, 58–66.

Landau, R. and Werner, S. (2012) Ethical aspects of using GPS for tracking people with dementia: recommendations for practice. *International Psychogeriatrics*, **24**, 358–366.

May, C., Gask, L., Atkinson, T. *et al.* (2001) Resisting and promoting new technologies in clinical practice: the case of telepsychiatry. *Social Science and Medicine*, **52**, 1889–1901.

McCormack, B. and McCance, T. (2010) *Person-centred Nursing: Theory, Models and Methods*. Wiley Blackwell, Oxford.

Morris, M.E., Adair, B., Ozanne, E. *et al.* (2014) Smart technologies to enhance social connectedness in older people who live at home. *Australasian Journal on Ageing*, **33**, 142–152.

Mort, M., Roberts, C., Pols, J. *et al.* (2015) Ethical implications of home telecare for older people: a framework derived from a multisited participative study. *Health Expectations*, **18**, 438–449.

Nieboer, M.E., Hoof, J. van, Hout, A.M. van *et al.* (2014) Professional values, technology and future health care: the view of health care professionals in The Netherlands. *Technology in Society*, **39**, 10–17.

Niemeijer, A.R., Depla, M.F., Frederiks, B.J. and Hertogh, C.M. (2015) The experiences of people with dementia and intellectual disabilities with surveillance technologies in residential care. *Nursing Ethics*, **22**, 1–14.

Nussbaum, M. (1999) *Cultivating Humanity*. Harvard University Press, Harvard.

Pols, J. (2012) *Care at a Distance. On The Closeness of Technology*. Amsterdam University Press, Amsterdam.

Roberts, C. and Mort, M. (2009) Reshaping what counts as care: older people, work and new technologies. *European Journal of Disability Research*, **3**, 138–158.

Schermer, M. (2014) Zorg op afstand; Zet goed leven centraal, in *Een verkenning van de grenzen, Etische overwegingen bij Zorg op Afstand*. Provincie Utrecht.

Simons, H. and McCormack, B. (2007) Integrating arts-based inquiry in evaluation methodology: opportunities and challenges. *Qualitative Inquiry*, **13**, 292–311.

Sparrow, R. and Sparrow, L. (2006) In the hands of machines? The future of aged care. *Minds and Machines*, **16**, 141–161.

Suter, P., Suter, W.N. and Johnston, D. (2011) Theory-based telehealth and patient empowerment. *Population Health Management*, **14**, 87–92.

Todres, L., Galvin, K.T. and Holloway, I. (2009) The humanization of healthcare: a value framework for qualitative research. *International Journal of Qualitative Studies on Health and Well-Being*, **4**, 68–77.

Zimmerman, M.A. (1995) Psychological empowerment. Issues and illustrations. *American Journal of Community Psychology*, **23**, 581–599.

Zwijsen, S.A., Niemeijer, A.R. and Hertogh, C.M.P.M (2011) Ethics of using assistive technology in the care for community-dwelling elderly people: an overview of the literature. *Aging and Mental Health*, **15**, 419–427.

6 A Participatory Approach to Person-Centred Research: Maximising Opportunities for Recovery*

Larry Davidson, Chyrell Bellamy, Elizabeth Flanagan, Kimberly Guy and Maria O'Connell

What's going on with these types of people? Do you really want to know? ... Do you really want that information? And if people can feel that vibe from a person, they will open up so much more. And I believe you all will have so much material that you can really do something with. (Participant in a study by Flanagan et al., *2012)*

INTRODUCTION

The comment above was made by a woman in a participatory study focusing on the subjective experiences of persons diagnosed with schizophrenia at the end of an hour-long qualitative interview that had been conducted with her by a person with her own history of mental illness and recovery. Even though participants in this study had received an average of over 20 years of treatment for a serious mental illness, several divulged important information to the interviewer that they then followed with the comment: 'But you're the only person I've ever told'. What kind of information is this woman referring to, why hadn't that information been shared with anyone else over the previous 20 years, and why did she, and other participants, 'open up so much more' to this interviewer? These are the types of questions we will be answering in this chapter as we take up the development and use of a participatory approach in research on serious mental illnesses and in the design and evaluation of interventions to promote recovery.

In order to maximise persons' opportunities for recovery in clinical practice, care needs to be person-centred, along with being strength-based, culturally competent and trauma-informed (Davidson et al., 2009).

But what about research? Is it possible to conduct research in a person-centred fashion? And, if so, how might such research also contribute to maximising opportunities for recovery, both for those directly involved and for future generations who may benefit from the findings generated by it, i.e. the 'material' that the field 'can really do something with'? Over

* Acknowledgement: work on this chapter was supported by the funding provided by a Eugene Washington PCORI Engagement Award made to Dr Davidson by the Patient-Centered Outcomes Research Institute, an independent, non-profit research institution authorised by the US Congress.

the last two decades, we have developed an increasingly participatory and person-centred approach to psychiatric research that we have found to do just that.

This chapter describes the evolution of this approach, offering a few examples of different ways in which persons in recovery can be involved in conducting a person-centred approach to research that generates clinically relevant findings aimed at improving the quality of care and enhancing those outcomes that matter most to the people of concern – in this case, persons living with serious mental illnesses and their loved ones.

HOSPITAL OR COMMUNITY?

The first series of studies that we conducted focused on the role of the psychiatric hospital in the treatment, lives and recovery of these persons. We began these studies as the last round of de-institutionalisation was taking place in the USA, 40 years after the legislation initiating the depopulation of mental hospitals had been passed. At that time, in 1954, approximately 500 000 people were living in state hospitals across the country, posing an increasing financial burden on state budgets while providing largely custodial care for the people in the hospitals. Not only had hospitals built for hundreds of patients been expanded to house thousands, but the 100-year-old buildings were requiring costly renovations and repairs as well as on-going maintenance. By the 1990s, many of these hospitals had closed, or at least been significantly downsized, with the total number of residents nearing 50 000; a 10-fold decrease. Still, over 50 000 persons remained and states were actively trying to move those they could into community placements. This provided the context for our first effort to include persons with serious mental illnesses in research; at first as primary stakeholders – that is, as the people who will be the most directly affected by the results of the research, but who, in the past, had seldom been included in it in any substantive way.

In retrospect, this degree of involvement may seem trivial to some readers. At the time, however, it was initially regarded as frivolous and foolhardy. Of the literally hundreds of articles and books published about de-institutionalisation since the 1960s, we could find only a handful of studies that had elicited the perspective of those persons living in the hospitals themselves (Davidson et al., 1996). When we embarked on such a study ourselves, initially we were met with much scepticism, as if a person living with a serious mental illness would either not have a perspective on the issue at all or, if they had one, would be unable to articulate that perspective in ways others could understand or find useful. What we found instead was that these people had much important information that they appreciated having the opportunity to share and that the picture they painted was more complicated than that of a simple either/or question of where would they rather live, the hospital or the community? As it turned out, they had many serious issues on their minds beyond the pressing question of where they slept at night.

For the first study, we interviewed a total of 12 people between 6 and 9 months following their discharge from a long-term stay at the state hospital (the average duration was 10 years) (Davidson et al., 1995). Much to our initial surprise – and despite the fact that all participants voiced a preference for living in the community – their narratives were much more focused on the similarities, rather than the differences, between the two settings. In both settings, their lives revolved around limited social interactions against a backdrop of loneliness, isolation and despair. Of life in the hospital, for example, one woman said:

> Well, [I'm] at the canteen every day. My mother sent money, [so I'd] buy cigarettes, buy candy, buy coffee, buy gum, buy soda, buy tea, buy soup, saltines and cheese and ham and bagels, and, you know, buy food and listen to the music. (Quoted in Davidson et al., 1995)

Another participant described his life in an apartment in the community in similar terms:

I just sit at my table and drink soda or water and smoke and listen to the radio and get a few memories by listening to the music. Or occasionally I'll turn on the TV and watch a pretty good movie. And we get together and sometimes we go out [to] McDonald's and have a little bite to eat. (Quoted in Davidson et al., 1995).

This gentleman also poignantly articulated the sense of hopelessness and helplessness that was shared by all of the participants when he said:

Well, there's nothing really out here for me...I'll say a prayer, say God help me or heal me or take [me]. But it hasn't worked so far...It's hard for me to concentrate, and sometimes when someone says something I may get a reminder of the past. I live in the past. Every day is the present, but it holds nothing for me. As far as the future, I have no future worth mentioning... I know I'm going to die mentally ill. I don't know what else I'll die from physically, but as far as hopes, I don't see any hope...I fear that I'll get sicker and linger on and suffer more than I'm suffering now. (Quoted in Davidson et al., 1995).

Another somewhat surprising finding in this study was that the participants found a greater sense of safety in the community than in the hospital. One concern that had been voiced by mental health providers was that the urban, inner city environment to which people were returning might render them vulnerable to victimisation; a concern that certainly has been shown to be credible in other studies published since then which have shown that persons with serious mental illnesses are at increased risk for victimisation (e.g. Sells *et al.*, 2003). Within the context of this study, however, participants were more likely to describe the hospital as unsafe due to the unpredictable behaviors of both staff and fellow patients. As one man said: 'I was afraid that if I made one wrong move someone would knock me down'. When asked if he felt safe in the hospital, another man noted: 'Not really, 'cause you never knew who was going to hit you or if you'd wind up in restraints' (quoted in Davidson *et al.*, 1995).

In the end, participants favoured the community due to the sense of privacy, freedom and safety it afforded and because they were closer to family and their neighborhoods of origin – the places where they were from. They stopped short of describing any sense of belonging in or to the community, however, accounting for why they did not participate much in community activities by saying things like: 'I wouldn't fit in because I'm bipolar' (quoted in Davidson *et al.*, 1995). In addition to the isolation and despair they described, participants also found it more difficult to receive adequate medical care in the community; a finding that has since been replicated and shown to account for a significant proportion of the discrepancy in lifespan among this population (Parks *et al.*, 2006; Laursen, Nordentoft and Mortensen, 2014).

However, perhaps most importantly, what we learned from this study was that persons with serious mental illnesses had a very different perspective from those people making the decisions about their care and their day-to-day lives and that, when asked, they could provide very clear and compelling accounts of the impact of those decisions and the terms in which they viewed and valued their own experiences. As has since been amply documented in terms of the discrepancies in valued outcomes between healthcare providers and their patients (e.g. Lieberman *et al.*, 1996; Fischer, Shumway and Owen, 2002; Say and Thomson, 2003; Kiesler and Auerbach, 2006), our participants were less concerned with the either/or question of *where* they lived and were more concerned with *how* they lived, resulting in a more complex and multidimensional understanding of what each setting offered and what each setting lacked. While the community was closer to home and family and offered safety, privacy, and freedom, in its current form it left people feeling terribly alone, hopeless and helpless, and at risk for serious medical conditions and complications that contribute to premature mortality. Above and beyond resolving the particular, and perhaps simplistic, question with which we began, the picture people painted of their daily lives provided valuable guidance for further policy and programme development efforts to decrease social isolation and increase hope, efficacy and overall wellness.

Building on the lessons learned in this first study, we next applied this approach of stakeholder involvement to the problem of inpatient recidivism; the phenomenon of persons with serious mental illnesses cycling through numerous brief admissions and readmissions to community hospitals – a phenomenon characterised by providers and policy makers as that of 'revolving door patients' (e.g. Cotterill and Thomas, 1993; Pfeiffer, O'Malley and Shott, 1996). Despite a body of empirical evidence that suggests that the major factors predicting readmission are social and environmental, as opposed to personal or clinical, in nature (e.g. Green, 1988; Kent, Fogarty and Yellowlees, 1995; Kent and Yellowlees, 1995; Appleby *et al.*, 1996; Klinkenberg and Calsyn, 1996), the conventional approach to preventing rehospitalisation at the time focused on early identification and prevention of relapse. It was based on the clinical assumption that patients ended up back in the hospital due to exacerbations of their disorder and, using a deficit-oriented model of care, focused almost exclusively on monitoring for and treating the signs and symptoms of the disorder. At our particular academic medical centre, such an approach had been attempted but had not borne much fruit. We were not experiencing any success in encouraging people to monitor their signs and symptoms, not a single patient had attended a relapse prevention group following discharge from the hospital, and people continued to be readmitted at high rates within 90 days of discharge.

It was at this point that the administration agreed that we should ask the patients themselves for their perspective and input. Similar to the study above, we identified and interviewed 12 persons with serious mental illnesses who met the eligibility criteria for having had multiple hospital admissions within the previous year (Davidson *et al.*, 1997). Similar to the study above, we discovered important aspects of the participants' everyday lives that helped us to understand their multiple readmissions and which generated useful implications for practice, both of which we describe briefly below. However, in this study we also learned two new and valuable lessons. First, we learned that we had not known what questions to ask prior to actually engaging with this population and, second, we learned that the persons most directly involved – our participants – had their own valuable ideas about ways to improve practice. It did not need to be up to us to interpret and address the implications of the research for developing new interventions on our own, but the participants' role could be expanded to include soliciting their input and feedback regarding what we might do in the future as well.

The first and most striking finding of this study was that the acute inpatient unit was viewed very differently from the long-stay hospital described in our initial study above. We learned this lesson in two ways, first by asking the wrong questions and second by being flexible enough in our approach to allow us to make mid-interview corrections when we realised our mistakes. The focus of the interview was initially on what the person and the mental health centre staff could do to prevent readmissions. We did not realise prior to trying out the interview how this focus reflected our own agenda, the agenda of the mental health centre and system, and not necessarily that of the people being served. We learned this when we tried out the questions and were responded to with blank stares and quizzical looks. For those participants who responded at all, the gist of their response was: 'Why would you try to keep me out of the hospital?' When this line of thinking was pursued, participants were able to say that they were sick and that they thought the hospital was for people who were sick, so why would you try to keep a sick person out of the hospital; wasn't that what it was there for? And when asked, in a related vein, if there was anything they could do on their own to cope with their illness or improve their lives, they replied that they were already doing their best just to get through life day-to-day. As one participant said, all I can do is to 'just take my medicine and pray'. Another said: 'I can't answer that one. Nobody knows the future, you know. I could be talking to you today and end up back in the hospital tomorrow' (quoted in Davidson *et al.*, 1997).

Against this backdrop of disability and powerlessness, more than half of participants described the hospital as providing a 'vacation' from their lives on the streets or being alone in shelters or their apartments. Even one person who had been hospitalised against his will described his most recent stay in the hospital as a 'forced vacation'. Another said: 'It's like a vacation, you take some time out ... in a place where there is privacy and there is care and there are lots of people to listen to you' (quoted in Davidson *et al.*, 1997). In addition to the attention they received, participants described the hospital as offering safety, privacy, food and respite, suggesting just how difficult and elusive these aspects of life can be to obtain or achieve on their own in the community. As one example, sleeping in a bed with only one or two strangers in your room offers more privacy and safety than sleeping on a cot 12 inches away from strangers on both sides of you in a room that holds 30. Most important to the participants, however, was the care and concern they experienced while in the hospital. For instance, as one person said: 'You see at home you don't have to listen to nobody but yourself. When you come into a hospital it's different. You're around a whole bunch of people that care about you' (quoted in Davidson *et al.*, 1997).

So significant was this sense of caring that they received in the hospital, and so much a contrast did it provide to their isolated lives in the community, that participants did not view readmissions as problematic at all (as had the administration). In fact, some talked about how much better each admission became over time as the staff came to know them and as they became more used to the unit routine. As summed up by one man: 'The first time I was scared, the second time I had been here before and I knew what to expect, the third time it was like coming home again. Everyone was like greeting me at the door ... The third time was the best I think' (quoted in Davidson *et al.*, 1997). Another person put the contrast in starker terms, describing how outside of the hospital no one cared whether he lived or died, while in the hospital every morning a doctor came to his room to ask him how he had slept the night before. Rather than sharing the administration's concern that they were coming back to the hospital too often, these participants saw the hospital as providing a beacon of care, safety and nourishment for both the body and the soul in the midst of a largely heartless and hopeless landscape. No wonder that one participant stated that: 'I felt that I had a better chance living here than living in society' (quoted in Davidson *et al.*, 1997).

Other than viewing the staff as caring and interested in their welfare, though, participants described 'treatment' in the hospital to be largely unresponsive to the concerns they had in the community. One participant compared participating in treatment groups to participating in the research interview itself, as he said: 'Well, it was something like this where they ask you questions. It was like going to school [and] I passed ... I passed with flying colors. Everybody loved me after I left that place' (quoted in Davidson *et al.*, 1997). A female participant expressed a similar sentiment about her treatment team and the unit milieu when she said:

I loved it, because they knew what was wrong with me, and they were trying their best to help me; so I agreed with everything they said ... There were a lot of meetings, a lot of doctors, you know, doctors come around every morning to talk to you to see how you're doing. You get your levels, your levels are one to five, one, two, three, four, five; when you come in you're a one. To go, the goal is to leave as a five. (Quoted in Davidson et al., 1997)

This kind of attention to unit routines and participation in treatment groups did not appear to translate into meaningful connections for people between treatment and coping on a day-to-day basis, however. When speaking of issues such as symptoms, medication, or coping with daily life, participants unanimously described the staff as the only ones who carried responsibility for understanding their illness and promoting their recovery. Agreeing with staff, attending groups and answering questions, obtaining a level 5, none of this had anything to do with addressing the illness or improving their actual lives.

Involving participants in coming up with ideas for improving practice thus required a different tack than a typical practice or quality improvement project. At a loss for how to prevent readmissions or enhance treatment, participants nonetheless had useful ideas for how to make life in the community more liveable, thereby lessening the degree to which hospitalisation offered a more preferred alternative. Discussions with these participants, as well as with other mental health service users who had been hospitalised previously but were now leading meaningful lives in the community, suggested several directions for programme development to address the restoration of community life. As we already had learned from our first study, we needed to find a way to address the social isolation and loneliness people were experiencing in the community. We needed to find some way to offer them a sense of belonging and mutual concern outside of the hospital that paralleled the feeling of camaraderie and care they had experienced inside the hospital. We needed also to find a way to overcome the feelings of powerlessness, fatalism and apathy people experienced in relation both to their mental illness and their lives in general. We needed to find a way to instil hope and provide concrete evidence of their own agency and efficacy, of the role they could play in promoting their own recovery. Lastly, we needed to address the pervasive disconnection they experienced between treatment in the hospital and life in the community, finding ways to demonstrate to people that treatment could be of direct benefit to them in addressing their day-to-day challenges and improving their daily lives. The ENGAGE intervention that we developed in collaboration with these stakeholders is described in detail in Table 6.1 below.

These interventions were provided within the context of twice-weekly groups co-led by a clinician and a peer staff member along with a weekly social and recreational outing in which people participated without the clinician. Groups and outings included food and were oriented to exploring and finding viable avenues for community living. The clinician group leader also consulted with participants' outpatient providers about the participants' daily life struggles and their goals for treatment in order to increase the responsiveness of care. Within the context of a randomised trial in which this intervention was compared to care as usual and a conventional skill-based group intervention, the ENGAGE intervention was found to increase the use of mental health services (Figure 6.1), the collaborative and culturally responsive nature of care (Figure 6.2), and social functioning (Figure 6.3), while also decreasing alcohol use (Figure 6.4) among persons with serious mental illness and co-occurring substance use disorders with histories of multiple hospitalisations. Unfortunately, as has been the case with assertive community treatment and other models of intensive clinical care, when the ENGAGE intervention ended, its positive effects on service use also disappeared, as also seen in Figure 6.1. Nonetheless, the intervention has helped to spawn a new generation of peer-delivered services and supports, and a new level of involvement of people in recovery in research, to which we turn next.

Table 6.1 ENGAGE intervention.

Social isolation to social support	Demoralisation to self-efficacy	Disconnection from, to engagement in treatment

1. Assist group members to engage in social connections with other group members.
  a. Encourage members to share their experiences of social disconnection and isolation.
  b. Assertive community outreach.
  c. Provide transportation to groups for 3 months, and then as indicated.
  d. Maintain twice-weekly personal contact with members for 3 months, then as indicated.
  e. Assist members to get half-price bus passes.
  f. Encourage members to accompany each other to assist in learning bus routes.
2. Facilitate and encourage specific acts of mutual support and reciprocity among members.
  a. Encourage expressions of caring, camaraderie, and friendship among group members.
  b. Assist members to recognise and respect social cues and personal boundaries in their interactions.
  c. Three home visits are made to new members by peer support staff to provide home supplies and lists of local community resources, and to help members fill out personal interest inventories.
3. Facilitate local community outings and activities with group members.
  a. Provide planning, financial support, and transportation for once-weekly, local community outings led by peer support staff.
  b. Enhance members' independence, and familiarity and connections with affordable, local community activities and resources.
4. Create and maintain group celebrations.
  a. Assist members to celebrate milestones in recovery and maintaining community tenure.
  b. Enhance members' connections with seasonal rhythms, and with local events and celebrations.
5. Facilitate participative group planning to increase members' personal investment in upcoming meetings, activities and events.
	1. Assist group members to recognise and share problems they face, and changes that occur.
	  a. Encourage members' expressions of hope in the possibility of change and recovery.
	  b. Encourage members to recognise and share downward and upward social comparisons.
	  c. Encourage members to share their struggles with constricted resources and help them apply for needed assistance.
	2. Facilitate participatory decision-making and planning among group members.
	  a. Help members to recognise how their actions impact on the group and other members.
	  b. Help members make specific, constructive plans for unstructured time, such as weekends.
	  c. Strengthen experiences of mutual accountability and responsibility among members.
	3. Provide individually tailored, flexible support to group members experiencing crises.
	  a. Increase engagement and contact intensity.
	  b. Provide transportation to extra outpatient appointments and intermediate care facilities.
	  c. Provide clinicians with assessments of functional deterioration and crisis intensification.
	  d. Advocate for interdisciplinary team meetings to plan special support and outreach efforts.
	4. Facilitate the emergence and recognition of group members' natural interests.
	  a. Encourage members to state preferences and interests in participatory planning for meals, community outings, and in group celebrations.
	  b. Encourage members to initiate activities with others who share their interests.
	  c. Recognise members' particular strengths, skills and natural leadership roles in activities.
	  d. Recognise and encourage members to share ways their interests motivate initiative, and enhance engagement in community activities.
		1. Help group members to face symptoms and destructive patterns of relating as these become evident in the lived interactions of the group.
		2. Help group members recognise changes and improvements in their symptoms and problems.
		3. Connect group members with abstinence-based self-help groups for substance use.
		  a. Support members' engagement in these groups by rewarding it with positive group recognition.
		  b. Encourage members to connect with sponsors.
		  c. Assist members with transportation if indicated.
		  d. Facilitate group celebrations of turning points and milestones in recovery.
		4. Assist group members to experience themselves as active partners in their care.
		  a. Help members to recognise their fears of medication side effects and stigma.
		  b. Train members in using the person-centred care planning workbook and offer to act as advocates on their behalf in care planning.
		  c. Assist members to face honestly struggles between acquiescence and compliance.
		5. Assist group members to connect experienced stress with symptom exacerbation.
		  a. Facilitate problem solving to help members reduce the impact of some stressors.
		  b. Assist members to find activities and other strategies for reducing experienced stress.
		6. Advocate for flexible, collaborative care planning with outpatient clinicians and other service agencies.
		7. Provide outpatient clinicians with information about members' daily lives and environment; cultural/racial/ethnic/gender/religious identity; and functional disabilities and strengths.
		8. Consult to outpatient clinicians regarding frustration and demoralisation around group members' continuing difficulties.

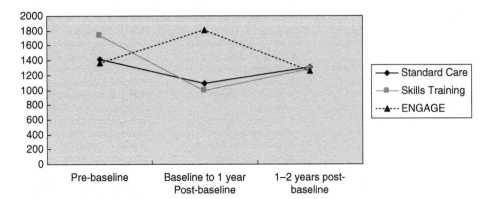

Figure 6.1 Total duration of services during first and second year post-baseline. ENGAGE participants have a significantly greater increase in time spent in services from before baseline to the first year after baseline than Standard Care (est. = –765.26, P = 0.04) and Skills Training (est. = –1183.19, $P<0.001$).

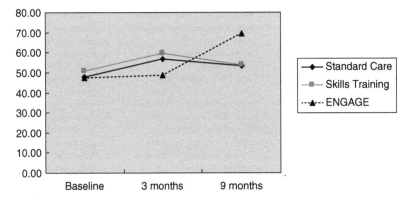

Figure 6.2 Collaborative and culturally competent services (CCCS). ENGAGE participants demonstrated significantly greater improvement in CCCS scores from baseline to 9 months than Standard Care (est. = –16.36, P = 0.04) and Skills Training (est. = –19.04, P = 0.01).

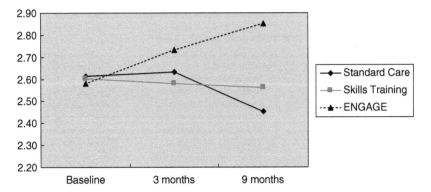

Figure 6.3 Social functioning. ENGAGE participants have a significantly greater increase in social functioning from baseline to 9 months than Standard Care (est. = –0.43, P = 0.01) and Skills Training (est. = –0.31, P = 0.05).

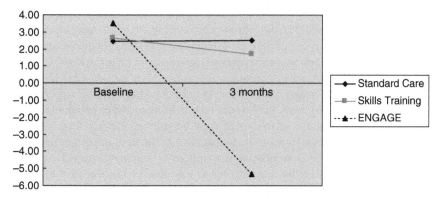

Figure 6.4 Problems with alcohol in last 30 days. ENGAGE participants demonstrated a significantly greater reduction in problems with alcohol use in the past 30 days from baseline to 3 months than Standard Care (est. = 8.84, P < 0.001) and Skills Training (est. = 7.89, P < 0.001).

PERSON-CENTRED CLINICAL RESEARCH

Having learned that we did not always know how best to frame our central research focus (e.g. living a better life in the community as opposed to keeping people out of the hospital) or precisely what questions to ask, we next increased the degree of stakeholder involvement to include persons in recovery in framing the research focus and developing the interview questions. Wondering also if we might receive different responses based on who was conducting the resulting interviews, we also began to train stakeholders to conduct qualitative interviews using a phenomenological, experience-based, approach.

One of the first studies to deploy this approach was led by Elizabeth Flanagan, PhD, focusing on how the subjective experiences of persons diagnosed with schizophrenia compare to the descriptions of these experiences offered in the *Diagnostic and Statistical Manual of Mental Disorders* (*DSM*), 4th edition, text revision (APA, 2000). One rationale for this study was that while the *DSM* claims to base diagnosis on the signs and symptoms of the various mental illnesses, these criteria have been defined and classified by clinicians and clinical investigators who have only mediated access to the experiences of the people living with these conditions themselves. No one had bothered to actually ask the people who presumably would know these conditions best, i.e. have the most direct and intimate familiarity with them, what these experiences had involved for them (Flanagan, Davidson and Strauss, 2010). In bringing together a research team that included a person who had been diagnosed with schizophrenia for over 25 years and another person in recovery who was trained to conduct qualitative interviews with others diagnosed with this condition, we were able to begin to explore the degree to which the *DSM* criteria for schizophrenia reflected these persons' own experiences as lived, and described, by them (Flanagan *et al.*, 2012).

In addition to exploring how the *DSM* reflects some, but not all, of the experiences of persons diagnosed with schizophrenia, this study taught us several important lessons, both about psychopathology and about clinical research. It was from the data collected for this study that we derived the quote with which we opened this chapter, for example. To be eligible for this study, participants had to have received over 20 years of psychiatric treatment associated with a diagnosis of schizophrenia based on *DSM* criteria. The central focus of the interview was on their experiences associated with having this condition, once again based on the criteria outlined in the *DSM*, 4th edition, text revision. So, participants were asked, for instance, about their experiences of delusions, hallucinations, thought disturbances and disorganised behaviour. Each term was accompanied by its description in the *DSM*. Conventional expectations of persons with schizophrenia, and reasons given for why they have yet to be involved in the *DSM* workgroups, are that they would deny having these experiences or at least lack insight into having them, they would be too disorganised or paranoid to be able to provide coherent or accurate descriptions of their experiences, and/or they would be too overwhelmed by negative symptoms to participate at all. The first, important finding of this study was that none of these conventional assumptions or arguments turned out to be true. Instead, and as mentioned in the introduction to this chapter, several of the participants remarked that the rich, descriptive responses they gave to the interviewers' questions included information they had never shared with anyone else before. As suggested by the woman we quoted at the opening, it appeared that once a certain 'vibe' was felt from the interviewer, participants were able to 'open up' and talk about what was really 'going on' with them in ways they had not done previously.

How are we to understand this? We suggest that these responses the participants gave, which we summarise below, were made possible by a combination of the questions asked and the credibility, openness, accessibility and skill of the interviewer. The interview differed from a diagnostic evaluation by adopting a person-centred and open-ended approach, following each inquiry about a specific sign or symptom with the seemingly simple question: 'What has that been like for you?' That is, after asking whether or not the participant has had delusions, has held beliefs that others did not hold, the interviewer then asked (following an affirmative response): 'and what has that been like for you, to have such beliefs?' Or, in the case of hallucinations, after establishing that a participant has heard voices that other people did not hear, the interviewer then asked: 'What has it been like to hear those voices?' To which the participants responded with a variety of answers, including: 'It's scary. It gets scary. I don't want to hear voices'; 'It's embarrassing'; 'Very scary, very scary. It's a terrible feeling. I wouldn't wish it on my worst enemy. Yeah, it's very scary, real scary'; 'It's like hell, a little bit of hell. The more voices I hear, the more I'm in hell'; and 'It's strange … It's hard. It gets to you. You're thinking 'I'm the only person that hears voices. Nobody hears them' (quoted in Flanagan *et al.*, 2012). Such responses were just the tip of the proverbial iceberg, though, and were followed by more elaborated narratives of how these experiences affected them and their daily functioning; one aspect, in particular, which they appeared not to have shared much with others.

We had already encountered this sentiment in the ENGAGE study described previously, in which participants had talked about the bleak and persistent realities of their daily lives and how their experiences of treatment had not been responsive to these struggles. In this study led by Flanagan, we were learning about some of the more hidden, or at least less obvious, reasons for this chasm between the realities of everyday life and the content of participants' treatment sessions. Before turning to how these experiences affected day-to-day life and functioning, we pause to consider this chasm and its possible contributors. What light did the participants shed on this issue? One person said:

> *The doctors don't fully understand, they really don't. A lot of people don't fully understand. Number one, they think you're crazy, you know, like a lot of people I talk to. And I'm not a crazy person, but it's the point that we go through things that people can't even fully imagine, you*

know. We can tell you certain things, but it's almost like saying you've never been to prison. I can tell you about prison. I can tell you everything. But until you experience being in prison, it's a whole different story. And that's how it is with this sickness thing that, you know, we're diagnosed with.

Another participant said:

I get kind of down a little bit. It makes me tear. My eyes get a little watery sometimes, because like my wife said, I feel too different. I feel weird, you know. You feel like an outcast. You feel like an alien, like not an alien, you know, like a monster alien, but like a place you don't belong. People don't fully understand you. They don't. You have nobody you fully can really talk to about whatever the thing is you're going through, because they're so more into what they're doing instead of more of what you're going through.

Most practitioners, as well as most other people in the person's life, haven't had the kind of (psychotic) experiences the person has had and do not see it as part of their responsibility to take the time to try to imagine what it might be like for this person to have to deal with these experiences, largely on their own. And, again often, when they take the risk of trying to share these experiences with others, rather than becoming concerned or curious, these others most often dismiss them, and their experiences, as being 'crazy'.

In contrast to the conventional clinical impression that persons with schizophrenia are not socially attuned to the affect or intentions of others, the participants in this study appeared to be very attentive to the attitudes and behaviours of other people, including but not limited to the clinicians providing their care. It was then on this basis that they actively chose what to tell to whom, complaining for the most part, however, that there was really no one in their lives to whom they could talk to about these most distressing, and, as we shall see, disabling, experiences.

The following are examples of how this was expressed:

'It's very frustrating. It's very frustrating, because you don't really know who to talk to about it. I try to talk to my doctor...the psychiatrist that I see every two weeks. We sit down, and she is a nice person. But the more you talk to them, the more they want to go up on your medication. I mean, what happened to just talking to the person and trying to find out what it is first?'

'Well, I don't say it to them, tell them that's going on. I don't want them to look at me like I am nuts. I mean, you know, I'm not nuts.'

'I'm embarrassed, I don't want people to tell there's something wrong with me. I know there's something wrong with me that I'm going through because they're not going through it, so obviously it's something wrong with me.'

'Most times I try not to even comment on it because if I say something they're just going to look at me like I'm nuts anyways.'

'I don't go there with people because it would be a waste of time and energy. Then they'll just look at you like you're even more of a kook, so I just don't.'

'I got to the point where I said I'm not going to talk to anybody about it. Unless I know someone that can really understand, which I mean nobody could, so I just kept it to myself.'

'But you're the only person I've ever told. I don't really tell my doctors that, because they'd probably really put me on more medication. So I ain't telling nobody nothing.'

We included so many of these quotations, but not nearly all, in order to give the reader an impression of how widespread this response of shutting down and withdrawing was amongst the participants in this study. Not only is it important to understand that this is one common way in which persons diagnosed with schizophrenia may deal with the stigma and misunderstandings associated with having a mental illness, but it is also important to note how concerned these individuals are with how they are seen and treated by others.

In reading these passages from the interviews, we can all readily understand how people might choose not to share certain information with others whom they have come to expect to view and dismiss them as strange, nuts or crazy. This has been far from obvious, however, as the conventional stereotype of persons with this diagnosis is that they are incapable of reading and responding appropriately to social cues and that they become indifferent to others, withdrawing into themselves as a consequence of the negative symptoms core to the illness process. These interviews present a very different picture that has very different implications for practice. In fact, what these interviews suggest is that at least some people diagnosed with schizophrenia have an exquisite sensitivity, a kind of radar, for detecting other people's attitudes and actions and that much of their more overt presentation reflects an attempt to keep their own experiences of the psychotic dimensions of the condition secret. They have withdrawn at least in part in self-defence, to protect themselves against further rejection and disappointment; a stance eloquently described by Patricia Deegan, PhD, a national leader of the service user movement in the USA who was diagnosed with schizophrenia in her youth. She writes:

> The professionals called it apathy and lack of motivation. They blamed it on our illness. But they don't understand that giving up is a highly motivated and goal-directed behavior. For us, giving up was a way of surviving. Giving up, refusing to hope, not trying, not caring; all of these were ways of trying to protect the last fragile traces of our spirit and our selfhood from undergoing another crushing. (Deegan, 1994, p. 19)

Given the open-ended nature of the questions, the credibility, trustworthiness, and skill of the interviewer, and their considerable courage, participants in this study were able to give us a glimpse behind this protective screen. What they described was a complex and interacting array of intense emotional reactions, both to the anomalous experiences they were having (e.g. hearing voices, holding beliefs others did not endorse) and to the fact that other people did not share these experiences, leaving them feeling that they were alien or that there was 'something wrong' with them. In addition to the fear and embarrassment already noted, having these experiences was distracting, confusing and exhausting, getting in the way of the person being able to pretend to be, to 'pass' as, 'normal' (Flanagan and Davidson, 2009). Confirming the validity of these findings, Richard Weingarten, another service user leader in the USA, wrote similarly of his own struggles. He wrote:

> Aggravating matters more is the painful knowledge that you can't talk to anybody about these things. Not only are these things hard to talk about, but if you admit to having any of these kinds of problems you are likely to get puzzled looks or face immediate and often final rejection. Most people will put you in the category of 'crazy' or 'looney tunes' or 'nutcase' or something similar. So to avoid this kind of abuse you are forced to hide or conceal your thoughts and feelings from others, and then ultimately from yourself, which only serves to worsen the situation... This is why persons with mental disorders are often passive, withdrawn and avoid human contact. They are engaged in an inner struggle they can't express and which consumes them... The invisibility of [this] struggle...and the isolation that results is what makes their situation so tragic. (1994, p. 374)

WHAT (ELSE) PERSONS IN RECOVERY CAN CONTRIBUTE

Over the last decade or so, it has become increasingly clear that persons in recovery can play as many roles in, and make as many contributions to, research as anyone else. As more clinicians and investigators living with mental health conditions have disclosed that they are in recovery (e.g. Corrigan, Larson and Michaels, 2015), and as more persons enter into recovery and become interested in contributing in various ways to research, the boundaries between those with and those without mental illnesses have become fluid and permeable, if not dissolved altogether. As a result, persons in recovery have joined research teams in numerous ways beyond simply consulting on what questions to ask or conducting qualitative interviews. At the same time, some funders of healthcare research grants (e.g. the Patient-Centred Outcomes Research Institute in the USA) have begun to insist on the involvement of primary stakeholders in all phases of the research process, from serving as consultants to convening their own research teams as principal or lead investigators.

The degree to which, and how, persons in recovery contribute to research reflects more the degree to which they are interested in, and have been prepared, to do so than anything about their psychiatric condition. Avenues for involving persons in recovery have expanded to include individuals who initially know little about the nature, conduct or purposes of research. They might start out by participating on a Community Advisory Board, for which they meet with other stakeholders and members of a research team to guide the development and implementation of a specific project. Or they might start out collecting focus group or interview data that would then be analysed by other members of the team. Successes in these endeavours may then lead them to obtain training in data analysis as well as data collection, or perhaps to return to school to obtain their own formal research training and credentials. To prepare interested parties for taking on a variety of these roles, we have developed a stakeholder network that educates persons in recovery and their loved ones about all aspects and phases of research and evaluation – from study design through dissemination – and then trains and supports them in taking on the roles of their choice (Davidson *et al.*, 2014).

Not surprisingly, one area in which the contributions of persons in recovery have been particularly important has been in the rapidly expanding area of peer support. We define peer supporters as people who have experienced a mental health condition and are either in or have achieved some degree of recovery. In their role as peer supporters, they use these personal experiences of illness and recovery, along with relevant training and supervision, to facilitate, guide and mentor other persons' recovery journeys by instilling hope, role modelling recovery, and supporting people in their own efforts to reclaim meaningful lives in the communities of their choice. Given this definition, it should be rather straightforward how and why research teams investigating this topic need to include persons with lived experience of recovery, as they are the experts when it comes to turning their own life lessons into valuable assets for others. This is only one example of the application of the motto of the disability rights movement of 'Nothing about us, without us' to the realm of psychiatric research and practice.

We have now been developing and studying peer support services for almost 20 years. Readers who are interested in the details of these various studies are referred to the body of published work that has been produced to date (e.g. Davidson *et al.*, 1997; Chinman *et al.*, 2001; Rowe *et al.*, 2007; Tondora *et al.*, 2010; Sledge *et al.*, 2011; Davidson *et al.*, 2012), as getting into the specifics of each study would take us beyond the scope of this chapter. In general, though, what we have learned from these studies is that persons in recovery functioning as peer supporters can maximise opportunities for the recovery of those they are supporting by instilling hope, by decreasing demoralisation, substance use, and the use of costly acute care services, and by increasing engagement in outpatient services, sense of well-being and activation for self-care.

CONCLUSION

We have learned first-hand that having people with first-hand experience of the health condition being researched, and/or of the treatments being offered, can increase the quality, relevance and utility of the findings being generated. Comprising a research team made up of healthcare professionals, persons in recovery, and family members – all of whom may wear more than one of these hats at any given time – we have witnessed the mutual learning that takes place when stakeholders from different perspectives are brought together with the common purpose of improving the lives of persons with serious mental illnesses. Consistent with the emphasis on collaboration in the delivery of person-centred care, we have found collaboration to be equally crucial to the conduct of person-centred research, expanding the benefits for maximising opportunities for recovery from those offered to users of mental health services to those being made available to persons taking on a variety of roles in carrying out research and evaluation studies, from consulting, to designing, implementing and disseminating, to leading their own teams through all phases of the process. In this case, though, the benefits extend beyond those individuals and families receiving care to all of those affected by these conditions, the broader research field, and the community as a whole.

REFERENCES

American Psychiatric Association (2000) *Diagnostic and Statistical Manual of Mental Disorders*, 4th edition, text revision. psychiatry.org (accessed 1 February 2017).

Appleby, L., Luchins, D.J., Desai, P.N. *et al.* (1996) Length of inpatient stay and recidivism among patients with schizophrenia. *Psychiatric Services*, **47**, 985–990.

Chinman, M.J., Weingarten, R., Stayner, D. and Davidson, L. (2001) Chronicity reconsidered: improving person-environment fit through a consumer-run service. *Community Mental Health Journal*, **37**, 215–230.

Corrigan, P.W., Larson, J.E. and Michaels, P.J. (eds) (2015) *Coming Out Proud to Erase the Stigma of Mental Illness: Stories and Essays of Solidarity*. InstantPublisher.

Cotterill, L. and Thomas, R. (1993) A typology of care episodes experienced by people with schizophrenia in an English town. *Social Science and Medicine*, **36**, 1587–1595.

Davidson, L., Bellamy, C., Guy, K. and Miller, R. (2012) Peer support among persons with severe mental illnesses: a review of evidence and experience. *World Psychiatry*, **11**, 123–128.

Davidson, L., Hoge, M.A., Godleski, L. *et al.* (1996) Hospital or community living? Examining consumer perspectives on deinstitutionalization. *Psychiatric Rehabilitation Journal*, **19**, 49–58.

Davidson, L., Hoge, M.A., Merrill, M. *et al.* (1995) The experiences of long-stay inpatients returning to the community. *Psychiatry: Interpersonal and Biological Processes*, **58**, 122–132.

Davidson, L., Ridgway, P., O'Connell, M.J. and Kirk, T.A. (2014) Transforming mental health care through the participation of the recovery community, in *Community Psychology and Community Mental Health: Towards Transformative Change* (eds G. Nelson, B. Kloos and J. Ornelas). Oxford University Press, New York. pp. 90–107.

Davidson, L., Stayner, D.A., Lambert, S. *et al.* (1997) Phenomenological and participatory research on schizophrenia: recovering the person in theory and practice. *Journal of Social Issues*, **53**, 767–784.

Davidson, L., Tondora, J., O'Connell, M.J. *et al.* (2009) *A Practical Guide to Recovery-Oriented Practice: Tools for Transforming Mental Health Care*. Oxford University Press, New York.

Davidson, L., Weingarten, R., Steiner, J. *et al.* (1997) Integrating prosumers into clinical settings, in *Consumers as Providers in Psychiatric Rehabilitation* (eds C.T. Mowbray, D.P. Moxley, C.A. Jasper and L.L. Howell). International Association for Psychosocial Rehabilitation Services, Columbia, MD. pp. 437–455.

Deegan, P. (1994) A letter to my friend who is giving up. *The Journal of the California Alliance for the Mentally Ill*, **5**, 18–20.

Fischer, E.P., Shumway, M. and Owen, R.R. (2002) Priorities of consumers, providers, and family members in the treatment of schizophrenia. *Psychiatric Services*, **53**, 724–729.

Flanagan, E. and Davidson, L. (2009) Passing for 'normal': features that affect the community inclusion of people with mental illness. *Psychiatric Rehabilitation Journal*, **33**, 18–25.

Flanagan, E., Davidson, L. and Strauss, J.S. (2010) The need for patient-subjective data in the *DSM* and *ICD*. *Psychiatry*, **73**, 297–307.

Flanagan, E., Solomon, L.E., Johnson, A. *et al.* (2012) The experience of schizophrenia in relation to its depiction in the *DSM-IV*. *Psychiatry*, **75**, 375–386.

Green, J. (1988) Frequent rehospitalization and noncompliance with treatment. *Hospital and Community Psychiatry*, **39**, 963–966.

Kent, S., Fogarty, M. and Yellowlees, P. (1995) A review of studies of heavy users of psychiatric services. *Psychiatric Services*, **46**, 1247–1253.

Kent, S. and Yellowlees, P. (1995) The relationship between social factors and frequent use of psychiatric services. *Australian and New Zealand Journal of Psychiatry*, **29**, 403–408.

Kiesler, D.J. and Auerbach, S.M. (2006) Optimal matches of patient preferences for information, decision-making and interpersonal behavior: evidence, models and interventions. *Patient Education and Counseling*, **61**, 319–341.

Klinkenberg, W.D. and Calsyn, R.J. (1996) Predictors of receipt of aftercare and recidivism among persons with severe mental illness: a review. *Psychiatric Services*, **47**, 487–496.

Laursen, T.M., Nordentoft, M. and Mortensen, P.B. (2014) Excess early mortality in schizophrenia. *Annual Review of Clinical Psychology*, **10**, 425–448.

Lieberman, J.R., Dorey, F., Shekelle, P. *et al.* (1996) Differences between patients' and physicians' evaluations of outcome after total hip arthroplasty. *Journal of Bone Joint Surgery in America*, **78**, 835–838.

Parks, J., Svendsen, D., Singer, P. and Foti, M.E. (2006) *Morbidity and Mortality in People with Serious Mental Illness*. National Association of State Mental Health Program Directors, Alexandria, VA.

Pfieffer, S.I., O'Malley, D.S. and Shott, S. (1996) Factors associated with the outcome of adults treated in psychiatric hospitals: a synthesis of findings. *Psychiatric Services*, **47**, 263–269.

Rowe, M., Bellamy, C., Baranoski, M., *et al.* (2007) Reducing alcohol use, drug use, and criminality among persons with severe mental illness: outcomes of a group- and peer-based intervention. *Psychiatric Services*, **58**, 955–961.

Say, R.E. and Thomson, R. (2003) The importance of patient preferences in treatment decisions—challenges for doctors. *British Medical Journal*, **327**, 542–545.

Sells, D., Rowe, M., Fisk, D. and Davidson, L. (2003) Violent victimization of persons with co-occurring psychiatric and substance use disorders. *Psychiatric Services*, **54**, 1253–1257.

Sledge, W.H., Lawless, M., Sells, D. *et al.* (2011) Effectiveness of peer support in reducing readmissions among people with multiple psychiatric hospitalizations. *Psychiatric Services*, **62**, 541–544.

Tondora, J., O'Connell, M., Dinzeo, T. *et al.* (2010) A clinical trial of peer-based culturally responsive person-centered care for psychosis for African Americans and Latinos. *Clinical Trials*, **7**, 368–379.

Weingarten, R. (1994) The ongoing processes of recovery. *Psychiatry*, **57**, 369–375.

7 Co-Creating Flourishing Research Practices Through Person-Centred Research: A Focus on Persons Living with Dementia

Kirsti Skovdahl and Jan Dewing

INTRODUCTION

Given demographic trends in many countries, it is likely that more people taking part in research will be older and will have multiple conditions that require researchers to be more thoughtful and creative about the best ways to enable positive and meaningful engagement in the research process. Persons with diminishing cognition, despite being a group that is increasing in size, have scarcely been heard; not something we can ignore in healthcare research. For this reason, in this chapter we have chosen to focus on persons living with dementia. Persons with dementia are most likely to be older, or ageing more rapidly, and have progressively diminishing cognition.

This chapter will focus on generic principles that can enable researchers to design or co-construct with persons with dementia more person-centred and therefore more contextually relevant methods and processes when engaging in some sort of participatory research connected to living with dementia. We recognise that participatory research is a continuum and participation will vary according to a number of factors, of which just a few, maybe, relate to how the person manages the consequences of dementia and other health and social needs. In this chapter, through sharing generic principles, we intend to:

1. Illustrate how philosophical perspectives shape research design in dementia care.
2. Discuss the principles underpinning participatory research.
3. Share a few of the key challenges for us as person-centred researchers.

BEGINNING WITH THE VOICE OF PERSONS WITH DEMENTIA

We want to begin by turning to and drawing directly on the life expertise of persons living with dementia and what they have to say about involving persons living with dementia in research. However, we are mindful that those we draw on are not speaking for all persons with dementia. A subgroup of the Scottish Dementia Working Group (2014) has developed

Person-Centred Healthcare Research, First Edition. Edited by Brendan McCormack, Sandra van Dulmen, Hilde Eide, Kirsti Skovdahl and Tom Eide.
© 2017 John Wiley & Sons Ltd. Published 2017 by John Wiley & Sons Ltd.

six principles for researchers wishing to involve persons with dementia in their research. The first principle is making sure persons with dementia and nominated others understand the research; the second principle requires researchers to value the experience and expertise of the person with dementia. We feel that this should be the first principle. Principle 3 sets out guidance about the best environments for persons with dementia so that they can actively be involved. We find this a challenging principle as many environments in which research takes place may not be enabling or person-centred. Principle 4 asks researchers to keep their language and communications simple. The fifth principle requires that researchers know something about dementia and about persons with dementia. This principle is vague in that it is not specific about how either dementia or the person with dementia needs to be understood. Principle 6 concerns keeping to 'dementia time' and being sensitive about how the person with dementia experiences time and time management. These core principles challenge researchers across all disciplines to reconsider how people with dementia are involved and valued in research as well as how knowledge is constructed in dementia research.

Swaffer (2016), coming from a different, perhaps more radical perspective, suggests that many, although claiming to want persons with dementia to have their rights, have in fact become used to having all the power:

> *What appears to be happening between people without dementia and those of us speaking up and living beyond dementia, is that the co-dependence many family care partners and society relied upon – and indeed, have gotten very used to – is disappearing, and our rights to autonomy and equality is being demanded.*

In fact, Swaffer (2016) uses the term 'living beyond dementia' to highlight that persons living with dementia do not need to be exclusively defined by the dementia. It is not the totality of personhood or identity. This serves as a note of caution, if not a warning, for person-centred researchers to ensure that we really do consider how we go about extending invitations of inclusion, participation and ultimately collaboration to persons living with/ beyond dementia and to reflect on assumptions that can be made about a person with dementia that are more focused on the dementia than the person.

As persons living with and beyond dementia do become more actively involved in research, researchers need to correct or moderate tokenism, and reliance on the same few contributors. Tokenism is where one person with dementia is included or where the numbers of persons with dementia are significantly lower than the professional researchers and/or where the contribution persons with dementia are asked to make is minimal.

EVOLVING INCLUSION AND PARTICIPATION

When we consider research that has taken place to date we see a less than ideal narrative regarding inclusion, participation and collaboration (Murphy *et al.*, 2015). As an example, a systematic review within the dementia and dementia care fields of research (1980–2005) by The Swedish Agency for Health Technology Assessment and Assessment of Social Services (2005), shows that research had in general the following foci: during the 1980s, the focus in the research was mainly on how the condition and related 'diseases' affected the brain. In the 1990s, the main focus was on formal and informal caregivers to persons with dementia and the caregivers' needs for support and education. In 2005 it was suggested that two of the next narratives to emerge would be connected to diagnosis and 'challenging behaviours' by persons with dementia; both are currently trending very clearly in the research literature. The Behavioural and Psychological Symptoms of Dementia model (BPSD) needs to be critically challenged by any researchers with a person-centred perspective. This label has effectively medicalised and made abnormal almost all types of emotional and human behavioural responses in almost all situations once a person has a diagnosis of dementia. Cahill, O'Shea and Pierce (2012) comment that the use of proxy accounts began to be questioned when it emerged that these accounts differed significantly from the experiences of persons with dementia themselves. We have inherited decades of either leaving the person with dementia out of research or token and minimal participation. Additionally, we have seen the person presented in a particular and very limited way that is underpinned by a set of limited and damaging assumptions, values and beliefs about the relationship of cognition and dementia to personhood (Sabat, 2001; Post, 2006, p.231; Dewing, 2008).

In progressing person-centred research approaches with persons living with dementia, researchers can expect to encounter different values about how central the person with dementia can be in any research. Most often the pretext that it is unethical to include persons with dementia in studies due to the risk of upset or harm will be put forward. The view that it is more unethical not to include persons with dementia as participants or co-researchers may need to be introduced and justified. Being able to refer to similar research carried out by others in your network can offer decision-makers, especially those in ethics committees, some confidence to take what they see as a risky decision. Further, it is helpful to keep up-to-date with the calls from dementia activists regarding their 'right' to be included in research.

THE RESEARCH PARADIGM

At its simplest, a paradigm is a complex belief system that guides the way we are and how we do things in research; it can help researchers establish theoretically rigorous and coherent approaches (methodologies) and related sets of methods. Paradigms are influenced by differing sets of assumptions, values and beliefs about reality and about knowledge. Therefore, examining our personal values and beliefs alongside philosophical principles can enable a more rigorous appreciation of our belief systems and our understanding of reality as well as the type(s) of knowledge we draw on and generate through research. In the case of participatory research with persons living with dementia, examining what we believe about personhood in the presence of declining or changing cognition and capacity seems essential. If, for example, a researcher concludes that rationality is central to personhood, then it would follow that an individual with dementia would have lesser personhood as their decision-making capacity declined. This then implies there would be less need for the person with dementia to be regarded as an active knowledge creator and therefore less need for active participation. Whereas the researcher who believes that the essence of personhood is not primarily dependent on or even lies outside of rationality or external to the physical body, is more likely to base their research on principles that will maintain and even nurture personhood. This implies that the person with dementia would be actively welcomed to participate as they are valued as having a contribution to make however the world is perceived and experienced. We suggest that the type and amount of power and control exercised by the researcher is, in part, proportional to their own values and beliefs. The consequences of believing a person with dementia has lesser personhood, with a lower standing or status, are widespread in terms of how this flows into and through research over the last decades and it is something that person-centred researchers need to address.

Person-centredness can be found in many different and we argue, exciting, guises in most if not all philosophers' works. It is (hopefully) both a joy and challenge for many healthcare researchers to delve into major philosophical works, even if they lie outside the usual comfort zone. An added challenge for new researchers is that few researchers within dementia care research have really developed deep and coherent philosophical ideas, with perhaps for the exception of Hughes, Kontas and Sabat. The most influential thinkers can provide the cornerstones and foundations for healthcare research and help us frame our new knowledge more effectively. We, for example, are influenced by the ideas of the French phenomenologist Maurice Merleau Ponty (1908–1961), the feminist ethic of care (for example, Gilligan, 1982), the Jewish philosopher and existentialist Martin Buber (1878–1965) and the Danish philosopher and theologian Knud Løgstrup (1905–1981). Over and above theorising, person-centredness is a human ethical presence. Levinas (1916–1995) proposes a line of thought similar to Martin Buber's idea of 'I and Thou', but with the emphasis on a relationship of respect and responsibility for the other person rather than a relationship of mutuality and dialogue (Buber, 2004). According to Løgstrup (2007) our attitudes to the other person help us to determine the scope and hue of his or her world. We help to shape his or her world not by theories and views but by our very presence towards him or her. Herein lies the unarticulated demand of being a person-centred researcher; that 'We never have anything to do with another human being without holding some portion of his life in our hands' (Løgstrup, 2007, p. 2).

RELATIONSHIPS

Relationships are perhaps the most visible feature of the enactment of person-centredness in any context. There is a need to 'do' research in a way that enables the person with dementia to be an active partner in the relationship. To achieve this, we argue, is more about a way of being than it is about 'doing' the research. Inherent in this assumption is that the best interests of the person with dementia would always take priority over research method or data. This is possible even well into what is referred to as the later or advanced stage(s) of dementia, should the researcher be skilled enough to 'sway and move' in keeping with the way of being of the person with dementia. Creativity in how the processes are made real and meaningful may be called for. For example, the use of resources, conceived of as connection and communication props, can support better perception, memory recall and association. Photographs, videos and objects that can be touched and handled can enhance conversations about aspects of the research. For example, in one research project, one of us (J.D.) always wore the same bright primary coloured top/jacket and carried the same bag containing a range of props should they be needed.

Drawing on the McCormack and McCance model of person-centred practice (2016) there are five processes that need to feature in relationships between researchers and persons living with dementia:

1. Being sympathetically present.
2. Working with the person's beliefs (or working with what matters to the person in each relationship).
3. Engaging authentically.
4. Sharing decision-making (or enablement of expression of choices and preferences where decision-making capacity has significantly deteriorated).
5. Providing holistic care.

What each of these principles look like in action will vary according to the persons in the research (this includes the researcher) and the research. Further, the researcher will need to mediate or even buffer macros influences (McCormack and McCance, 2016) that may impinge on the research relationship.

CAPACITY AND PROCESS CONSENT

The matter of consent as a process is very closely woven into person-centred research. Trust and consent lie at the heart of an ethical relationship in all research. The Declaration of Helsinki (World Medical Association, 2000) states: 'For a research subject who is … mentally incapable of giving consent…, the investigator must obtain informed consent from the legally authorised representative in accordance with applicable law'. And in person-centred research, this extends beyond legal requirements. Clearly, for many persons with dementia, capacity to make decisions can alter and keeps altering. However, internationally, there is considerable variation in terms of how consent is handled and who can be an authorised representative, and indeed which research studies do and do not require formal ethics committee approval. Many countries also have legal statutes regarding capacity and decision-making. Despite this, some researchers (for example Fisk and Wigley, 2000; Dewing, 2002, 2007) argue that the legal requirements enabling authorised representatives to make decisions regarding participation in research (by the person with dementia) have the unintended consequence of excluding the person with dementia. It is possible for a researcher, while operating within the law, never to see or engage with the person with dementia until after ethical approval has been given and in effect the person with dementia has been 'consented' into the research. This feels inherently untrustworthy and in effect creates a moral distance or abyss. While Sherratt, Soteriou and Evans (2007) suggest that the wishes of individuals cannot be understood in all situations, and the views of those consulted cannot in all cases accurately reflect the views of the person they represent, the person-centred researcher needs to find ways of enabling inclusion. There should be an emphasis on the intrinsic value of each person with dementia, rather than on their decision-making competence. For example, some persons with dementia can respond to simplified information and informed consent forms, whereas others will require a more radical approach such as verbally giving consent. Then others, who will legally be outside formal informed consent, can still be engaged in a form of inclusionary consent process based on choice and experiential preferences that comes through from being in an authentic relationship (Dewing, 2002, 2007). We do not advocate the use of cognitive screening or assessment tools in research where this is not central to the research.

Voluntary, informed consent is based on the ethical ideal of protecting the individual's autonomy. On the other hand, it is inevitable that the researcher has the power over the situation in which the person may feel the weakest part. Persons with dementia, like all research participants, are dependent on the researcher to receive 'adequate' information about any project. Furthermore, the researcher is in a position of power. Every researcher has, in accordance with the ethical guidelines, the responsibility to pay attention to the participant's own best interests. Respecting every signal of (dis)stress and unwillingness to continue to participate in research are crucial. Consent for participation must therefore continue throughout the research process. It is challenging to know how best to do this as many researchers still do not detail their consent methods in reports and publications.

METHODS

Practically, in terms of research methods, it is challenging to meaningfully include some persons with dementia. This is particularly so, suggest Murphy *et al.* (2015), in the later stages of the condition where issues of consent, decision-making capacity and meaningful participation need to be addressed sensitively and creatively if inclusion is to be meaningful. It was assumed until recently, that persons with dementia did not make reliable interviewees and could not be relied on to provide valid research data (Smebye and Kirkevold, 2012). Having seen the emergence of the person with dementia in research slowly growing (for example, Downs, 1997), along with evolving and more person-centred values, beliefs and assumptions, the case for greater inclusion and participation is, argue Murphy *et al.* (2015), now compelling. We should remember that most persons with dementia are living in their communities and getting on with life and would make very suitable participants and perhaps co-researchers. Person-centred researchers still have much to do in terms of progressing more meaningful inclusion and participation by and with persons living with dementia. In particular, we need to focus more on how we go about achieving this intent throughout the whole of our research. The methods and the processes we employ as researchers are central to this.

Based on the principle that persons with dementia are embodied, self-creating social agents, the research methods designed by the researcher need to enable persons to be active participants and draw on the strengths and abilities they have rather than highlighting losses. This suggests a greater use of qualitative methods, where participants take a more active part. Even using qualitative methods, some further modifications may need to take place so that persons with dementia can engage as fully as possible. Researchers with limited skill and experience in adapting approaches and methods that enable participation need to ensure they access a more experienced researcher who can offer supervision and open up networks to connect with other person-centred researchers. A number of researchers have detailed dementia-friendly methods that have proven useful in different types of research. Looking back over research methods in one international peer-reviewed dementia-specific journal over the last 5 years, it seems that some form of interviewing remains the most popular or preferred method – at least by researchers. Making research methods dementia-friendly can include strategies such as establishing a person's strength of orientation and expressive capacity prior to any interview (Lloyd, Gatherer and Kalsy, 2006), very careful preparation of questions, timing of interviews, dealing with disruptions in orientation and attentions, and avoiding domination of the carer's perspective (McKillop and Wilkinson, 2004).

CONTEXTUAL FACTORS

There are, as we indicated at the start of the chapter, a few factors related to dementia that may impinge on the degree to which a person can participate in research. For the purposes of this chapter we will consider two factors; co-dependence and dependence on others and advanced dementia. Co-dependence and dependence on others is a feature of living with dementia that many persons with dementia contend with on a daily basis. Much research in the past replicated this taken-for-granted assumption. It was enabled to happen as carers were often present during interviews and it was their perceptions and experiences that tended to be captured (McKillop and Wilkinson, 2004). There are some particular opportunities and challenges associated with involving people with dementia in research in the long-term care context. To begin with, we cannot assume that persons will have an advanced dementia or that they are a captive participant as they have nothing else to do (Dewing, 2009). While many older persons living in care homes will have a more eclectic way of 'being in the world' (due to a more advanced dementia), many will have moved into a care home for other reasons and later acquired dementia.

We offer one scenario from our research that illustrates the context of being a person-centred researcher as well as illustrating the importance of relationships in engaging authentically. This example is from a study with persons with early dementia that focused on:

- The development of a passive position alarm in co-operation with persons with dementia, their spouses, and the company that developed the technique.
- The persons with dementia experiences and reflections from repeated participatory observations and dialogue in their home

In this study five persons with early dementia who had a desire and need to be outdoors and had wayfinding challenges, and her/his cohabiting family member, were included in a study that used participatory observations and repeated informal conversations in the person's home. The aim of the participation was to enable the person with dementia to share experiences about the passive positioning alarm used for being outdoors independently (for further information see Olsson *et al.*, 2012; Olsson *et al.*, 2013a). The researchers met the couples between five and seven times during a 3-month period. A co-observer participated to accompany and observe the person with dementia on his/her outdoor walk, while the other observer observed and had an informal conversation with the family member.

A significant focus was placed on building a naturalistic relationship and building trust and confidence together with the couples who participated in the study. At the start of the study, the researchers' roles were a barrier to building trustful relationships. What mattered most seemed to be our roles as registered nurses with experience of working within the dementia care field. Several participants expressed that this led them to feel they would be understood and that we were interested in them as persons and the development of support adapted to persons with dementia and not only interested in collecting data. 'Culture contingent rituals' also emerged as important in building relationships. For example, at first we declined coffee because we did not want to create extra work. We quickly realised that the serving of coffee was a natural part of welcoming guests into the home. After this, we accepted coffee and spent more time with everyday conversation before started talking about the research.

The participants shared that their contributions as research participants gave them a sense of purpose and usefulness and expressed their gratitude to be able to participate in the study. One of them also took the inititative to report her experiences in a blog, in newspapers and at a larger national conference. She expressed that she was proud to be an important part of developing support for persons with dementia in the future, through sharing her experiences as a person living with dementia.

This scenario shows us the meaning of involving persons with dementia as partners and resource persons in research and not only as 'participants' or 'informants'.

For researchers entering practice settings for any sort of intervention research, the organisational context and its culture will have an influence on the research in a number of significant ways and can be critical to the success of the research. Stockwell-Smith *et al.* (2015) identify four learning points for other researchers to include in planning their research:

1. Effective collaborative research requires an organisational [and workplace] culture that is open to research participation.
2. Invest early in relationship-building to establish strong buy-in from senior staff and identify influential champions to act as liaisons between the research team and key decision-makers.
3. Utilising an existing workforce is a potentially efficient means of delivering a research intervention
4. Output-based funding and workforce constraints greatly limit the capacity of service organisations to encourage staff involvement in research.

User involvement in the design and delivery of services and research is increasingly recognised as essential (NICE, 2013a, b). Persons with dementia are in a position to advise on the research questions that matter to them, and inform how the process and outputs of research can benefit those affected by the condition. Ultimately, we need to explore a whole range of possibilities including how persons with dementia can become researchers and equal members of a research team.

CONCLUSION

Although this chapter has focused on the importance of core principles to underpin participatory research with persons whose cognition is diminishing, we hope it has raised questions for person-centred research with other persons who have diminishing or an altered cognition. This can lead to uncertainties in the research design which while uncomfortable, can in the longer term contribute to the wider debate about what it means to be a person in a bio-technological and genetically engineered world. Core principles considered in this chapter include an examination and articulation of values and philosophical ideas on personhood in the context of living with or beyond dementia; person-centred relationships and designing and adapting methods and processes to enable persons with dementia to be participants. We have emphasised matters of embodied process consent as being central to (all) participatory researching. The chapter reminds us that the real challenge is not simply about how we involve persons with dementia, although that is often a real challenge for many of us, it is also about how persons with dementia can be enabled to construct and co-construct knowledge. It is this new knowledge that helps to shape and reshape our culture and ultimately will make a difference to lives. The delicate balance between protecting vulnerable individuals, recognising the importance and benefits to society of research and maintaining an individual's right to take risks including taking part in research is very real.

REFERENCES

Buber, M. (2004) *I and Thou*. Charles Scribner & Sons, 1937. Reprint. Continuum International Publishing Group, London.
Cahill, S., O'Shea, E. and Pierce, P. (2012) *Creating Excellence in Dementia Care, Dublin, Ireland*. DOH Dublin, Ireland.

Dewing, J. (2002) From ritual to relationship: a person-centred approach to consent in qualitative research with older people who have dementia. *Dementia*, **1**, 157–171.

Dewing, J. (2007) Participatory research: a method for process consent with persons who have dementia. *Dementia*, **6**, 111–125.

Dewing, J. (2008) Personhood and dementia: revisiting Tom Kitwood's ideas. *International Journal of Older People's Nursing*, **3**, 3–13.

Dewing, J. (2009) Making it work: a model for research and development in care homes, in *Understanding Care Homes: A Research and Development Perspective* (eds K. Froggatt, S. Davies and J. Meyer). Jessica Kingsley, London.

Downs, M. (1997) The emergence of the person in dementia research. *Ageing and Society*, **17**, 597–607.

Fisk, M. and Wigley, V. (2000) Accessing and interviewing the oldest old in care homes. *Quality in Ageing – Policy, Practice and Research*, **1**, 27–33.

Gilligan, C. (1982) *In a Different Voice: Psychological Theory and Women's Development*. Harvard University Press, London.

Lloyd, V., Gatherer, A. and Kalsy, S. (2006) Conducting qualitative interview research with people with expressive language difficulties. *Qualitative Health Research*, **16**, 1386–1404.

Løgstrup, K.E. (2007) *Beyond the Ethical Demand*. University of Notre Dame Press, Paris.

McKillop, J. and Wilkinson, H. (2004) Make it easy on yourself! Advice to researchers from someone with dementia on being interviewed. *Dementia*, **3**, 117–125.

Olsson, A., Engström, M., Skovdahl, K. and Lampic, C. (2012) My, your and our needs for safety and security: relatives' reflections on using information and communication technology in dementia care. *Scandinavian Journal of Caring Sciences*, **26**, 104–112.

Olsson, A., Engström, M., Lampic, C. and Skovdahl, K. (2013b) A passive positioning alarm used by persons with dementia and their spouses – a qualitative intervention study. *BMC Geriatrics*, **13**, 11.

Olsson, A., Lampic, C., Skovdahl, K. and Engström, M. (2013a) Persons with early-stage dementia reflect on being outdoors: a repeated interview study. *Aging and Mental Health*, **17**, 793–800.

McCormack, B. and McCance, T. (2016) *Person-centred Nursing and Healthcare: Theory and Practice*, 2nd edition. Wiley Blackwell, Oxford.

Murphy, K., Jordan, F., Hunter, A., Cooney, A. and Casey, D. (2015) Articulating the strategies for maximising the inclusion of people with dementia in qualitative research studies. *Dementia*, **14**, 800–824.

National Institute for Health and Care Excellence (2013a) NICE commissioning guide 48: Support for commissioning of dementia care. National Institute for Health and Care Excellence, London.

National Institute for Health and Care Excellence (2013b) NICE quality standard 30: Supporting people to live well with dementia. National Institute for Health and Care Excellence, London.

Post, S.G. (2006) Respectare: moral respect for the lives of the deeply forgetful, in *Dementia: Mind, Meaning and The Person* (eds J.C. Hughes, S.J. Louw and S.R. Sabat). Oxford University Press, Oxford. pp. 223–234.

Sabat, S.R. (2001) *The Experience of Alzheimer's Disease: Life Through a Tangled Veil*. Blackwell, Oxford.

Sherratt, C., Soteriou, T. and Evans, S. (2007) Ethical issues in social research involving people with advanced dementia. *Dementia*, **6**, 463–479.

Smebye, K. and Kirkevold, M. (2012) How do persons with dementia participate in decision making related to health and daily care? A multi-case study. *BMC Health Services*, **12**, 241.

Stockwell-Smith, G., Moyle, W., Kellett, U. and Brodaty, H. (2015) Community practitioner involvement in collaborative research. *Dementia*, **14**, 450–467.

Swaffer, K. (2016) Co-dependence and dementia. http://kateswaffer.com/2016/01/30/co-dependence-and-dementia (accessed 1 February 2017).

Swedish Council on Health Technology Assessment in Health Care (SBU) (2008) *Dementia – Caring, Ethics, Ethnical and Economical Aspects*. SBU report no 172E/3. SBU, Stockholm.

The Scottish Dementia Working Group Research Sub-Group (2014) Core principles for involving people with dementia in research: innovative practice. *Dementia*, **13**, 680–685.

World Medical Association (2000) *The Declaration of Helsinki*. www.wma.net/en/30publications/10policies/b3/ (accessed 1 February 2017).

8 Leadership Research: A Person-Centred Agenda

Tom Eide and Shaun Cardiff

INTRODUCTION

Leadership is important for the quality of healthcare services. Person-centred approaches to care delivery have been increasingly promoted in international policy and strategy. Person-centred values, like high quality care and respect for persons' integrity, dignity, security and rights are at the core of both national healthcare policies (NMHCS, 2009; HOD, 2015) and professional codes of ethics (ENDA, 2011; ICN, 2012). Despite this there is evidence of failings within healthcare systems that negatively impact on the care experiences of patients and staff (McConnell, McCance and Melby, 2015). In addition, contemporary healthcare systems are facing a series of challenges putting values at risk, such as a changing demographic and cultural landscape, a professional and leadership capacity gap, policy and organisational changes, and budget limitations and cuts. Realising person-centred values is a central leadership responsibility in healthcare. However, there is still little research in general on how to make values live in the organisation in general and on person-centred leadership in particular (Cardiff, 2014).

Over the last 20 years or so, considerable scholarly attention has been invested in the construct and conceptual framework of person-centred healthcare (Mead and Bower, 2000; McCormack, 2003; McCormack and McCance, 2010; Jakimowicz and Perry, 2015). However, person-centred leadership is still a new construct. There is little research in the field, no clear definition of the concept, and no consensus among scholars regarding theoretical foundation.

DEFINING PERSON-CENTRED LEADERSHIP

In this chapter we take a pragmatic stance, and propose to define *person-centred leadership* in healthcare quite broadly as leadership supporting, creating and securing person-centred values and practices. Person-centred leadership is ethical and teleological in nature, in the sense that the ultimate objective – *telos* – is a standard of care that ensures the patient or

Person-Centred Healthcare Research, First Edition. Edited by Brendan McCormack, Sandra van Dulmen, Hilde Eide, Kirsti Skovdahl and Tom Eide.

client is at the centre of care delivery (McCance, McCormack and Dewing, 2011), and is always treated with respect for the individual person's dignity, integrity and rights (ENDA, 2011; ICN, 2012; HF, 2014).

LEADERSHIP RESEARCH

In line with this definition, we propose to consider person-centred leadership *research* as basically normative and action-oriented, as research with the overall aim of supporting and improving the leadership practice of making person-centred values live in the organisation, i.e. enhancing the person-centredness of service designs, organisation cultures and – first of all – of healthcare practices, as experienced by patients, clients and other end users (service users).

There is a growing interest in the field of person-centred healthcare, but with a very few exceptions, the research on person-centred leadership is still scarce. In this chapter we will present two of our own research projects as examples of how to go about doing research in order to support and improve person-centred leadership practice. Both projects are participatory and action-oriented in design. Cardiff performed a study in a ward in a Dutch urban general hospital aimed at exploring and developing person-centred nursing leadership (Cardiff, 2014). Eide and colleagues undertook an educational design intervention in a medium size Norwegian municipality, aimed at creating a common vision of person-centred practice across 17 services and units (Eide *et al.*, 2014). Other recent studies have explored how situational and transformational leadership styles may influence the development of person-centredness in different care settings (Lynch, McCormack and McCance, 2011; Beckett *et al.*, 2013; Rokstad *et al.*, 2015).

THE TWO DOMAINS OF PERSON-CENTRED LEADERSHIP RESEARCH

These studies indicate directly or indirectly that the person-centred leadership and leadership research in healthcare has two main domains, the relational and the organisational. In the relational domain the leaders' primary concern is enabling associates to come into their own as persons and person-centred professionals. The term associate as a synoniem for 'other members of staff' reflects and reinforces the person-centred practice value of equality. In the organisational domain the leaders' primary concern is to create, develop and ensure person-centred services within their area of responsibility. The relational and organisational domains are two different, but interdependent areas of research, and can be studied separately or together.

The relational domain

While the ultimate person of focus may be the service user, on a day-to-day basis, practice leaders usually work more closely with colleagues/employees than service users. Therefore, the main person in question for the leader of a healthcare organisation or unit may be considered to be the employee. Accordingly, relational focused person-centred leadership research on this level should be guided by questions concerning leadership attitudes, approaches, styles, skills and roles. Research in this relational domain aims at improving the leader's person-centredness towards colleagues, and might be conducted for, with and/or on the employees.

The organisational domain

In the organisational domain the leader is responsible for delivering high quality, person-centred healthcare services. Many organisations have defined person-centred vision, mission and value statements. The main person in question in this domain is the individual service user. Accordingly, organisational focused person-centred leadership research should be guided by questions concerning the status of such espoused values and how leaders can or should go about making these values visible in the organisation. This might include studies of improvement strategies, interventions and processes on different levels and in different areas, like organisational structure, strategy, service design, organisational culture and systemic care practices. Leadership research in this organisational domain is conducted for the end user, and might be conducted on and with both leaders and employees.

THE THREE LEVELS OF PERSON-CENTRED LEADERSHIP RESEARCH

Person-centred leadership can be studied at different levels. The *telos* of person-centredness improvement can be found on all levels of the system. We can divide roughly between three main levels: the macro, meso and the micro level (see Figure 8.1). On the macro level of national healthcare systems, policies and programmes (the outer circle), we find the political leaders, laying down the structural, legal and financial premises for healthcare. On the meso level, we find the leaders of the healthcare organisations, like hospitals, municipalities and non-profit institutions, where national and local policies are operationalised. On the micro level we find the middle managers and leaders of the organisations' units and services, where person-centred care values are supposed to be brought into practice in practitioner–service user relationships.

The macro or system level

At the macro level the main research focus is on policy and system factors, such as national and international health politics and law. Research may also be guided by questions concerning political leaders' visions, priorities and rhetoric, including communication of political expectations concerning person-centred practice on the meso and micro levels. At this level research may apply methods and theories from different academic fields, including health law, sociology, political science, communication and organisation studies.

The meso or organisation level

At the meso level person-centred leadership research includes studying the role leadership plays at the top of the healthcare organisation in enabling processes that foster person-centred healthcare across services and units. Main areas of interest include organisational vision and values as well as interventions and processes aiming at shaping, supporting and improving person-centred leadership and practice at the micro level. On this level, research might be guided by questions concerning planning, organising and changing processes, informed by theories and methods from the broad field of management and organisation studies, including educational design research.

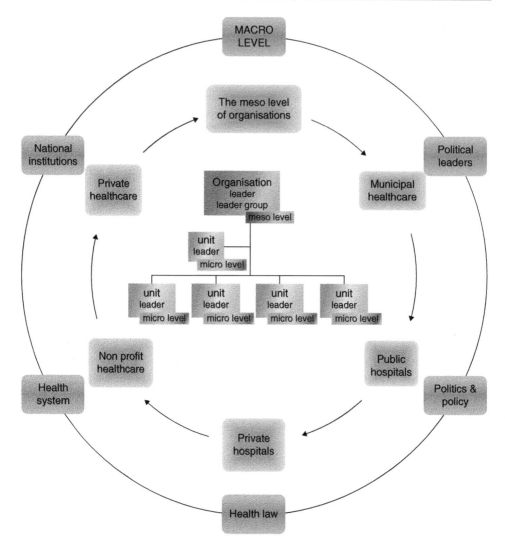

Figure 8.1 The three levels of person-centred leadership and leadership research. Leadership research may address both the relational and the organisational domain on each of these three levels. However, considering the overall aim of supporting and improving person-centred healthcare practice, research at the macro level might have a main focus on policy and system factors; research at the meso level on organisational strategies, designs and change; while research at the micro level most naturally might include a combination of relational and organisational aspects.

The micro or practice level

The micro level is where person-centred care is provided. Leadership research at this level supports and explores leaders' work with practitioners and support/administrative staff in co-creating service designs and organisational cultures that foster high quality, person-centred care practices. Person-centred practice may be characterised by four elements (Brooker, 2004, 2006): (1) valuing people and those who care for them; (2) treating people as individual persons; (3) looking at the world from the perspective of the person in question; and (4) recognising that all human life is grounded in relationships. Research on this level might be guided by questions concerning leadership roles and styles, service development and design, organisational culture and change, healthcare and quality improvement with a special focus on person-centredness. Studies might be informed by theories and methods from fields like health administration, healthcare management and organisation studies.

In the following section we will present examples of how person-centred leadership research on these three levels may be performed, starting with the macro level.

RESEARCH AT THE SYSTEM LEVEL

Questions of person-centred leadership at a macro level are mainly issues of political mindset and practice, of will and power to take the necessary initiatives and make the necessary systemic changes in order to ensure the interest, dignity and values of service users. Leadership research at this level may include questions of top leaders' mindset, positions and strategy plans concerning person-centredness within the healthcare system. This may concern questions of legislation, like the legal protection of patients' rights, autonomy and dignity (Molven and Ferkis, 2011), of health promotion on a system level (WHO, 2009; HSE, 2011), and of sociological and social science issues like the role of leadership in social justice, distribution of health and the justification and change of patterns of health and ill health.

Whether research at this macro level may be considered *person-centred leadership* research depends upon the leadership definition and theory used. There is little research of this kind available. There are, however, reasons for directing more research attention towards the political level, because the premises and possibilities for developing person-centred cultures and practices are influenced by politics and system design.

The case of Norway

The following example from Norway may illustrate a shift from a system-oriented towards a person-centred mindset at the macro level of politics and legislation.

Since before the turn of the century the Norwegian Board of Health Supervision has documented the failure of the healthcare system to meet individual service users' needs. As a response to this, a series of government initiatives were taken. We will mention four of these, representing a systemic turn towards ethical reflection and more person-centred organising and legislation.

National competence building in ethics

In 2007 the Government and the Norwegian Association of Local and Regional Authorities (KS) launched a national project on cooperation on building competency in ethics within the municipal health and care services. Within this initiative national and local educational conferences were held, handbooks of organisational ethics and ethical leadership were developed (Eide and Aadland, 2012; Eide, Landmark and Martinsen, 2015), and an annual, national 'ethics award' was established (2010). At the end of 2015 more than 240 of the 426 Norwegian municipalities have established various meeting places to strengthen expertise in ethics (Gjerberg *et al.*, 2014; Söderhamn, Kjøstvedt and Slettebø, 2014).

The coordination reform: proper treatment at the right place and right time

In 2009 the Minister of Health and Care Services, Bjarne Håkon Hanssen, launched the Coordination Reform and his vision of the health and care services: 'With smart solutions, patients will receive proper treatment at the right place and right time' (NMHCS, 2009). One could argue that this objective strengthens 'professional-centred care' rather than person-centred care. On the other hand, the shift in policy perspective is from the system towards the service user, and the white paper stresses the importance of patient autonomy, empowerment and shared decision-making. However, even though the *objective* of the Coordination Reform may be characterised as person-centred, the *measures* were mainly structural and systemic; 'the organisational development of services needs to undergo change, and frame-work conditions must be established that encourage the profession to cooperate better and provide services in accordance with political objectives' (NMHCS, 2009, p. 5).

The guarantee of dignity

In 2010 the Government drew up regulations on dignified care for older people that specify the municipalities' moral obligations (Guarantee of Dignity, 2010). The aim was to ensure that the older people are not neglected with regard to the overall activities of the nursing and care services. The regulations describe the values underlying care for older people and set out the measures to be implemented within the care services, such as appropriate and safe forms of housing, a varied and adequate diet, palliative treatment and a dignified death, pro-fessionally sound follow-up by doctors and other relevant personnel, conversations about existential questions, etc. The complaints and inspectorate authorities are responsible for ensuring that municipalities adhere to the *Guarantee of Dignity* (NMHCS, 2013, p. 40).

The Health Minister's project: to create the patient's health service

The final manifestation of a turn from a system-oriented to a person-centred mindset and practice at the macro level in Norway was when, in January 2014, the new Minister of Health and Care Services, Bent Høie, formulated his vision of future care, making *the patient's health service* his slogan: 'My project as Minister of Health and Care Services is to create the patient's health service. The patient shall be put at the centre, the waiting time shall decrease and the quality be increased' (Høie, 2014). This was followed up in the white paper *The Primary Health and Care Services of Tomorrow* (NMHCS, 2015), where the aim of person-centred services is clearly stated:

> *The Government seeks to promote patient-centred health care services. The needs of the patient must be the focal point of development and change in the health and care services. 'No decisions about me will be taken without me'. Achieving this will require change. (Introduction, p. 9)*

The Minister also calls attention to ethical reflection as a key indicator in quality improve-ment initiatives in the health and care services. In a series of speeches, he stressed the impor-tance of listening to service users, seeing them as whole persons, and reflecting on and with the service users on moral issues concerning health and treatment. Stressing the value of cooperative practices, good communication and having an authentic dialogue with service users, he repeatedly refers to an ethics award winning municipality having established ethics reflection groups where both service users and relatives were included. This illustrates what we mean by a person-centred mindset at macro level, namely combining person-centred strategic thinking and practice at the top level of leadership with a genuine concern for realising person-centredness at the service/end user level. This also demonstrates how leadership at a macro level may influence and support change at other levels.

There is a need for research on leadership from the top and to what degree and in which ways leadership and politics at a healthcare system level fosters and enables expectations of person-centred health and care services. Research with a person-centred focus at a macro level may be varied, from political science studies on systems of government, sociological studies of power in healthcare politics, studies of health law and implementation of legislation, to studies of political leaders' rhetoric, political discourse and text analyses of speeches, debates and documents, as exemplified in the fourth example here.

RESEARCH AT THE ORGANISATION LEVEL

Person-centred leadership at the meso level entails both *strategic leadership* aiming at developing person-centred attitudes and practices across services and units, as well as being a person-centred leader of middle managers, responsible for realising person-centred values and objectives in their own units and departments.

Person-centred leadership research at an organisational level might focus on top managers and the leader groups' leadership practice and style of interaction, as well as on their strategic work, such as development of organisational vision and values, strategic plans and processes for improvement of person-centred practice across services and units of the organisation as a whole.

Dependent on the objectives, person-centred leadership research at an organisational level can be more or less descriptive, normative and action oriented. Descriptive research might be driven by questions concerning the degree of person-centredness among the top management and/or questions concerning the status of person-centredness in the organisation's vision, mission and value statements, strategic goals and plans, and procedures for reporting. Normative research on this level may be driven by questions concerning how leadership practice ought to change in order to realise person-centred values in the organisation, while action-oriented research may be driven by questions aimed at generating knowledge necessary to support the process of implementing such change. Keeping in mind the distinction between research for, with and on persons, person-centred research on leadership at the meso level (like the macro level) will be *for* end users, often *with* (and for) leaders on different levels of the organisation, and sometimes also *on* (and with) the top managers and members of organisation management teams.

There is to our knowledge little research on person-centred leadership at the meso level. As an example of research at this level, we will report from a Norwegian participative action-research project aimed at creating a common person-centred focus across services and units in a municipal healthcare organisation.

The Dream project

In Norway, like in many other countries, primary care is mainly provided by the municipalities, who are responsible for putting macro level policy aims of person-centred practice into effect at an organisational level. Municipal health and social care services are complex organisations, often including a series of services and units of different kinds. There is often a lack of communication between services and units, and it is well documented that service users are often not treated as they should be. For instance, violations of security and rights quite frequently occur, often due to lack of coordination, information provision and user participation (NBHS, 2013), and are often due to leadership failure (NMHCS, 2015).

Vision and objectives

The Dream project was carried out in a medium size Norwegian municipality (70 000 inhabitants). The project was initiated by the Director of the municipality's health and social care organisation (HSO). The vision of the HSO was 'creating good days' for the individual service user. The overall objective of the Dream project was to make this vision come true, by improving person-centred practice and enhancing user value within and across services and units. The project comprised all 17 departments of the HSO, including the Director's staff, the R&D department (Figure 8.2) and two cooperative partners: the local hospital and the local NAV department (Norwegian Labour and Welfare Administration). Most departments consisted of several services and units. For instance, the eight local health and care services all included both home care and nursing homes, as well as assisted living services comprising of housing, day care and different support activities.

Dream was planned as a cooperative innovation project between the municipal HSO division and the Science Centre – Health and Technology of the local university college. 'Dream' is an acronym created from the name of the municipality (D) and the core values of the project (in Norwegian): reflection, ethics, workflow (*arbeidsflyt*) and participation (*medarbeiderskap*). The project was planned in three stages:

1. Creating a shared vision of person-centred practice across services and units.
2. Improving the person-centredness of service designs and practices.
3. Continuous service improvement aimed at 'creating good days'.

Here we report the first stage, with a focus on research and process design.

Participants and gatherings

The participants were two to three leaders or key persons from each service/unit, 38 persons in all (of about 120 leaders and other key persons in the HSO division). The participants were selected not primarily as representatives, but on the basis of their assumed interest in developing person-centred practice, their knowledge of the respective services and their potential for taking a leading role in implementing change.

Seven gatherings were organised during a period of four-and-a-half months (Figure 8.3). The overall aim was to develop a shared vision of the desired future concerning person-centred services (on a meso level) and to initiate local processes and service development projects (on a micro level) in order to make the future happen. The gatherings were held within the facilities of the municipality, and lasted for 2 days, except for the first and the third, which were one day only.

Action research design

The project had a participatory, educational action research design, consisting of lectures on lean and ethics, plenary search processes and local micro-processes and projects, developed and carried out by the participants and their associates in their own units. The process design

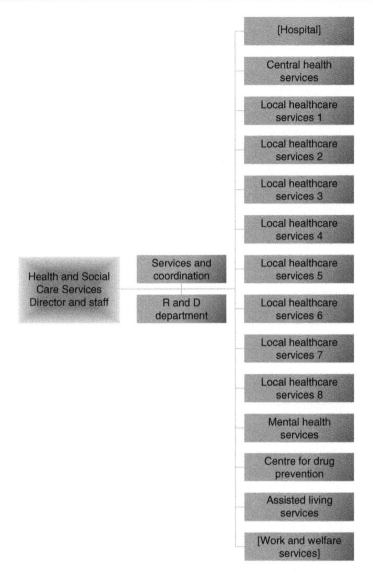

Figure 8.2 The Dream Project – participating departments and services.

was developed from different sources: lean innovation (Ries, 2011), organisational ethics (Eide and Aadland, 2012), literature and theory of mind (Eide, 2010; Kidd and Castano, 2013) and participatory action research (Reason and Bradbury, 2008). Inspired especially by search conference methodology (Emery and Purser, 1996; Levin, 2014) processes were designed in which the participants came together to find common ground on existing challenges and explore possible and desirable futures. Participation in the project was not about giving input to the top leaders responsible for strategy plans, but about taking part in developing a shared vision of the desired future (on an organisational level), and taking responsibility for developing and carrying out a plan together with their colleagues and associates to help realise the desired future (on the service level).

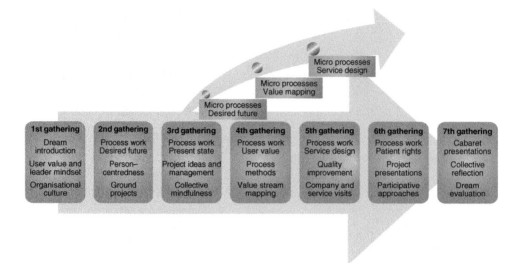

Figure 8.3 The Dream project – process development.

An educational design element was included (van den Akker *et al.*, 2006) in order to help the participants become empowered and build their competence for taking a leading role in initiating participatory processes and carrying out change projects within their own units. The educational part was focused on ethical leadership (Eide, van Dulmen and Eide, 2015) and lean leadership methodology (Liker and Convis, 2012), and included methods for participatory exploration of user values, mapping of values streams, identification of activities that do not create value for the service user (activities that should be dropped) and development of plans for making the future happen.

Data collection

Data were collected by participatory observation and questionnaires, as well as participants' written reflections (chart paper, digital notes), narratives, project plans and reports.

A note on lean

Here we refer to lean as an organisational philosophy built on the primacy of user value. Lean is controversial, often associated with downsizing and/or budget cuts. This is not the concept of lean applied here. Lean thinking starts with the concept of user value, meaning what the user actually needs and wants. It aims at developing strategies for bringing the organisation more in line with its core purpose, in this project to provide high quality, person-centred services. Lean methodology starts with identifying user value. It may proceed by value stream mapping, which here implies identifying work processes that provide value to the user (value stream) and how to sustain and improve the workflow and make it smooth. According to lean principles this is done by engaging every employee touching value streams, because those closest to practice are normally the persons best qualified to identify 'where the shoe pinches' and to see how the flow may be improved. To our knowledge – controversial as it may be – lean is the most consistent organisational philosophy when it comes to putting user value – person-centredness – first. Lean also offers a set of participative methods for critical organisation analysis from a user-centred perspective.

The researcher role

The researchers' role in the project was: (1) to develop the idea and design the processes together with the Director and staff members; (2) to facilitate the processes, including the creation of a safe, non-judgemental and creative space for collective exploration, reflection and learning; (3) to summarise the ideas voiced in plenary processes about the existing organisational functioning across services and units, especially about what should be kept, dropped and changed, to challenge the participants to continue and deepen their reflection and learning process, and (4) develop the educational design, including giving lectures on key issues.

Results

Little by little the participants built a community of mutual trust and creativity. The communication and learning across services and units were intensified. Increased knowledge of the other services was reported. Recognition of the necessity for smooth cooperation between services and units in order to enhance user value grew fast. Questions concerning user value and ethical issues were increasingly brought to the fore, and the concept of 'user value' became an integral part of the language used. Also, a change in the way problematic issues were voiced was observed, from a tendency to point to problems in other parts of the organisation to more open reflection on lack of flow and person-centredness within one's own services. These changes developed parallel with plenary reporting of local micro-processes. All 17 departments were engaged in micro-projects, some of them cooperation projects between several units and services, 12 projects in all. User value was investigated in different ways, such as questionnaires, narratives and interviews with patients.

The overall most important result of this first step in the Dream project concerned organisational culture, which included: (a) the development of a common focus on user value across services and units; (b) the enhanced openness of communication between the different parts of the organisation, and (c) the increased recognition of the role of each unit and the necessity of close cooperation in order to create workflow and user value. Three major issues, deemed critical across the services, seemed to emerge through the projects at a micro level: (1) the need to be listened to, (2) the wish to be informed and included in decisions, and (3) the requirement of receiving services when needed and promised. Also a series of other user needs were reported.

A fourth important issue emerging in the plenary sessions, explicitly addressed in the reflection and evaluation part of the last gathering, was the question of how to keep up the good work on enhancing workflow and person-centredness across services and units. Three assumed main success factors seemed to emerge from the discussions: (1) to continue the open dialogue across services and units, (2) to include more leaders in the process of competence building and change, and (3) to offer methodological support in developing and carrying out projects at a micro level. These results were communicated back to the Director and top leader group for planning the design of the next phases of the Dream project.

RESEARCH AT THE PRACTICE LEVEL

Leadership at the practice level entails the leading of others at the front-line of service provision, the point of contact between practitioners/members of staff and service users. While traditionally leadership is associated with hierarchical positions within an organisation, person-centred leadership at the practice level is relational, to some degree detached from management and hierarchical roles. From this perspective, leadership is 'a practice of caring for colleagues, enabling others to act, acknowledging and learning from one's mistakes and being emotionally authentic' (Binns, 2008), a relational practice through which social structures, conventions and practices can be maintained and/or transformed (Uhl-Bien, 2006). Also, person-centred leadership is basically ethical, a way of 'being and relating with others, embedded in everyday experience and interwoven with a sense of moral responsibility' (Cunliffe and Eriksen, 2011, p. 1432), the primary responsibility being to develop high quality, person-centred workplace cultures and practices.

Objectives of leadership research on this level might be to stimulate leadership reflection and improvement of person-centred practice. Research questions might focus on leadership *mindset and beliefs*, such as to what extent leaders' thoughts are dominated about organisational productivity and results, or about motivation and well-being of employees and quality of care for service users. Questions may also focus on leadership *attitudes and styles*, for instance whether the leaders are cooperative and participative, orientated towards 'power with' (coactive) employees and service users, or more authoritative and directive orientated, towards 'power over' (coercive) service users and employees. Research questions might also focus on leadership *skills, roles and strategies*, such as how leaders approach challenges concerning staff motivation or quality of care, for instance by balancing transformational and transactional approaches (Bass, 1990; Brown and Treviño, 2003).

By way of an example of research at this level, we will present a study aimed at exploring person-centred leadership as it was developed in collaboration with a nurse leadership team of a ward in a Dutch urban general hospital (Cardiff, 2014). In order to enable research done *with* rather than *on* leader participants and other stakeholders a participatory action research (PAR) was chosen. PAR entails the study of participant attempts to transform their social context for the good of all and in doing so co-produce emancipatory knowledge (Winter and Munn-Giddings, 2001). Participants in the action research team collectively inquire into the historical and contextual influences of their practice, regularly (self)critically reflecting on interventions, with an aim of acting appropriately. Researching change is carried out in the natural setting with varying degrees of participation, and traditionally has a design of an orientation phase followed by spirals of planning, acting, observing and reflecting/evaluating.

Action research for person-centred leadership

The study started in collaboration with a unit nurse manager and two charge nurses of a 24 bed acute care unit for older people in a 430 bedded urban general hospital in the Netherlands. Together they planned an orientation phase consisting of patient narratives about care, staff narratives about care and leadership, and overt participant observations of the unit culture. The findings were collectively reviewed with the whole team and issues for change identified.

Three issues formed the basis for action spirals. The first was the creation of biweekly reflective inquiries that created a communicative space for leaders to collectively, critically and creatively reflect on their practice (Cardiff, 2012). The second spiral entailed the development and implementation of a new nursing system based on the principles of primary nursing (Manthey, 2009). The third spiral entailed leaders facilitating short (15 minute) weekly storytelling sessions aimed at promoting a person-centred mindset among the care team members. Data were collected from six leaders engaged in operational leadership in both hierarchical and non-hierarchical leadership roles. Data collection methods included audio-recordings of the reflective inquiry sessions, workshops on visioning primary nursing and the primary nurse role, primary nurse evaluation meetings, workshops exploring the unit culture and leadership, as well as a staff questionnaire on perceptions of change within the unit. Participant observation by the researcher with post-observation interviews with the leader being observed, often accompanied by interviews with those they were leading during the observation period, also fostered insight into leadership in the public, private and personal sphere (Scouller, 2011).

When asked about the intent of their actions, participant leaders frequently used the phrase *'to enable people to come into their own'*. Consequently, the phrase became the theme describing the primary aim of person-centred leadership. It covers the moments where people were changing, shining, reaching their potential and/or being their authentic self. Moments when people felt good and things felt right. This is congruent with the emancipatory aim of critical social science (Fay, 1987) and person-centred practice (McCormack and McCance, 2010). Not only was there evidence of unit staff and culture coming into their own, participant leaders also experienced coming into their own and the researcher described how he too had undergone transformation for the better.

Five processes fostering relational connectedness between researcher and participants, as well as between leader and associates, were identified:

1. *Presencing* is a concept originally coined by C. Otto Scharmer to mean sensing, tuning in and acting from one's highest future potential (Senge *et al.*, 2005). Applied in person-centred thinking it means the relational process of 'being there' for the other person (McCormack and McCance, 2010). Beginning with unconditional openness and beneficent attentiveness with a sole aim of achieving relational connectedness, both parties can then decide if and how the professional can help (Klaver and Baart, 2011). As a researcher one might decide to be actively present, 'being with' and 'thinking with' leaders about interventions such as an education programme, rather than actively participating and 'doing for' the leaders.

2. *Communing*, means finding a common ground, building a shared vision and engaging in shared decision-making, and is also central to person-centred, participatory research. At times, the subject matter may be emotionally laden. Beginning with unconditional openness, beneficent attentiveness and an attitude of 'being there' for the other person is probably the best way of establishing such a common ground. In Cardiff's study, communing started during initial discussions between the researcher and participants about the study aim and design, and continued through until the results were published.

3. *Contextualising* entails the process of understanding participants as distinct persons embedded within a mix of (past/present/future) professional and social roles and contexts that (positively/negatively) influence their being, becoming and professional conduct. A person-centred researcher comes to 'know' each participant as an individual, and may

also use their own personal and professional knowledge to try to understand how context may influence participants and vice versa. Such understanding can help the researcher be creative in designing processes that help participants come into their own as person-centred leaders and professionals.

4. *Sensing* is the process of positioning self to actively and passively gather information (see, hear, feel) on where the other 'is at', and confirm interpretations. Sensing during overt participant observation, as well as during post-observation interviews, was central to making process decisions like supporting participant reflections on practice, diverging from planned actions, and creating space for participants to recuperate and/ or attend to pressing issues. Sensing may be considered the opposite of 'distancing for objectivity' (Grant, Nelson and Mitchell, 2008), often considered an academic ideal. However, sensing is in fact a way of remaining observant, reflexive and person-centred during the research process.

5. *Balancing*, means (morally) weighing (competing) needs of individuals, groups and self. Doing person-centred research we often find ourselves *balancing* the needs of the individual participant with those of other participants, as well as those of the research study and our own needs. Balancing implies genuine listening and dialogue – as prescribed by thinkers like Buber (1923/37), Rogers (1961), Freire (1970) and Habermas (1984). Ideal dialogue conditions are often difficult to achieve in everyday healthcare leader contexts (Grill, Ahlborg and Lindgren, 2011; Gillespie *et al.*, 2014). Balancing fostered authentic dialogues and helped ensure mutual recognition, respect and participation in decisions.

On the basis of this and other studies (Eide, van Dulmen and Eide, 2015; Rokstad *et al.*, 2015) we developed a conceptual framework for person-centred leadership research on the micro level (Figure 8.4).

The researcher role

The researcher, as leader of the research project, when doing person-centred leadership research at the practice level may be characterised by six elements, of which the first two are the most fundamental:

1. Being mindful that the research is conducted *for* the end user and – directly or indirectly – that the final goal of person-centred leadership research is to create a knowledge foundation for improving not only person-centred leadership, but also person-centred organisational culture and care practices.

2. Being mindful that doing research *on* leaders and staff members should imply treating participants as unique persons and ends in themselves, and – paraphrasing Kant's second formulation of the categorical imperative (Kant, 1785/2001) – never merely as research objects or means to an end. This implies authentically listening and being other-centred during the research process, as participants will sense whether or not they are being recognised, respected and understood.

3. Using a participatory approach, i.e. planning and conducting the research process *with* the leaders and other persons whose actions, attitudes and/or organisational design and routines are under study, and developing the specific research objective out of the convergence of the two perspectives – science and practice (Bergold and Thomas, 2012). This goes both for qualitative and quantitative approaches.

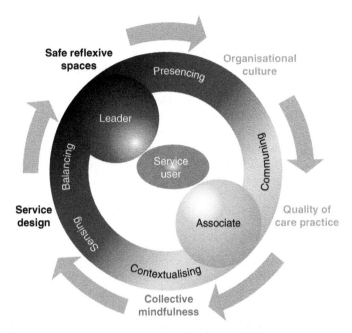

Figure 8.4 Person-centred leadership research on micro level. In the centre of the model we find the patient or service, in order to visualise that the final aim of person-centred leadership research is to create new knowledge in support of high quality, person-centred healthcare practice development. The two domains of leadership research, the relational and the organisational, are illustrated with two circles around the centre. In the relational domain, the inner circle, a leader's primary concern is the facilitation of associates, aiming to help them come into their own as person-centred professionals.

4. Fostering reflexivity, among participants in the organisation under study (Alvesson and Sköldberg, 2009) by creating safe, critical and creative spaces, as well as by the researcher self on their role and potential influence on others. This includes reflecting on the limitations of one's empathy and intrapersonal intelligence when trying to understand participants' emotions and perspectives, and of one's interpersonal intelligence when trying to foster participants' contribution and commitment.

5. Being courageous, open and patient during the research and reflection processes. This can help all 'roll with the punches' and 'ride the unexpected waves' of research life. Particularly in participatory research, participants may initially view the researcher as the expert and expect directive leadership, which would be contradictory to the principles of participation and gathering authentic data. A willingness to show one's vulnerability may foster relational equality and remove unfounded expectations that 'the researcher knows best' (Cardiff, 2014).

6. Stancing is the constant (re)positioning of self in relation to participants with an aim of maintaining/instigating momentum towards coming into one's own as a person-centred researcher/leader. Four basic leader stances were identified in Cardiff's study: leading from the front, the side-line, alongside and from behind. These stances could potentially be confused with those of situational leadership (Hersey, Blanchard and Johnson, 2001). However, the fundamental difference lies in leader intent. Situational leaders assess follower task competency and adjust their leadership accordingly.

Person-centred leaders are more holistic in their assessment of associate being, and are also concerned with enabling self-actualisation, empowerment and well-being. Leading from the front, the person-centred leader offers to role model and/or 'do for' the associate, whereas a situational leader would tell/instruct the follower. Leading from the side-line, the person-centred leader offers instructions and support, whereas the situational leader sells/persuades the follower to psychologically buy in to what the leader wants. Leading from alongside, the person-centred leader uses high challenge and high support in close (relational) proximity to enable associate self-directed action. Leading from behind, the person-centred leader steps back, creating space for the associate to act independently because they are competent and/or because this creates an opportunity for experiential learning.

The influence of the organisation

Many research methodologies and methods entail the study of participants in their natural setting, with inevitable consideration of *organisational culture* as 'the way things are done within the context' and the influence of social structures, traditions, values and beliefs. Social structures, conventions and practices are co-created by people in relation and simultaneously influence the way people interact. A researcher is often an 'outsider' and while this can be beneficial in unearthing implicit cultural phenomenon, researchers will also find themselves having to work with organisational cultural values and beliefs when planning and executing research activities. Cardiff found that awareness and responsiveness to workplace culture fostered participation and commitment. Many research activities were planned so as not to disrupt daily routines, or existent structures were slightly readjusted so that they became points for data collection. For instance, staff on the unit met daily from 13.45 to 14.15 hours to evaluate how each person was coping. It was agreed that one evaluation meeting per week could easily be reconfigured to form a storytelling session. Simultaneously, participation in the research activities, and reflecting on how the researcher interacted with participants, influenced how staff on the unit started to interact.

While intervention studies usually include learning activities, learning through change is fundamental to action research. With no formal practice developer/clinical educator positions on the unit of Cardiff's study, the participant leaders felt responsible for enabling staff learning. This was not limited to formal, structured learning such as a clinical education programme, but also included opportunistic, informal and unstructured learning within the workplace during a shift. Facilitated workplace learning can be both professionally and personally empowering (Merriam, 1996), especially when learners are invited and supported to review critically and creatively their personal being and that of the context (Snoeren, 2015). The outcome of *safe, critical and creative (learning) spaces* can therefore influence how people relate and existing relationships may form input for inquiry in such spaces.

The person-centred mindset encourages us not only to see the person before us but also those whose being may be affected by the decisions made. It is therefore appropriate that *differing stakeholder needs* within the contextual domain are given due consideration when relating with individual participants. As the participant leaders in Cardiff's study explored the concept of person-centredness and principles of action research, they consciously chose to create a think-group that represented as many stakeholder perspectives as possible when redesigning the nursing system. The primary nurses also collected data from different stakeholders when evaluating their role. Awareness of differing stakeholder needs also influenced how data were collected, for instance, verbal consent was obtained from those working with/being cared for by the primary nurses before participant observation started. Such consideration of differing needs fosters awareness of power within relationships.

Finally, to close this section on person-centred leadership at the practice level, and in particular, leading a (action) research project, we need to consider *evaluation systems*. Multiple methods were used in Cardiff's study to gather evaluative data for each action

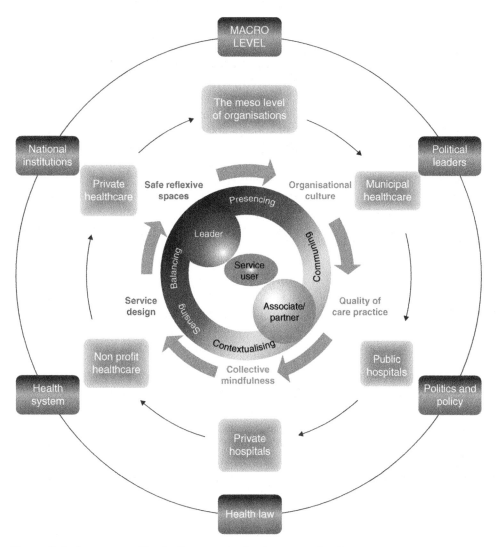

Figure 8.5 Person-centred leadership research – levels, areas and topics.

spiral, from multiple perspectives. Evaluative data were also collected continuously and/ or at multiple points throughout the study. The mutual influencing between the two domains was strong here as evaluations influenced how leaders related with staff, and the effects of these changes were captured in later evaluations. Evaluations were generally open in character, often asking for claims and concerns about that which was being evaluated so that issues for improvement could be identified and then possible actions. The openness helped ensure that which was felt to be of priority was attended to, and allowed evaluation of both products and processes. The same applied to the researchers' role and the influence of the research study on leader development.

TOWARDS A FRAMEWORK FOR LEADERSHIP RESEARCH

Many leadership theories and styles contain constructs congruent with a person-centred mindset and person-centred leadership. The leadership approaches most commonly attached to person-centredness are transformational leadership (Steiger and Balog, 2010; Lynch *et al.*, 2011; Beckett *et al.*, 2013; Cardiff, 2014), relational leadership (Uhl-Bien, 2006) and ethical leadership (Storch *et al.*, 2013; Eide, van Dulmen and Eide, 2015). However, most leadership approaches or theories highlight elements that are central also to person-centredness. Are there some distinctive features about person-centred leadership research compared with other kinds of leadership? Person-centred healthcare leadership research differs from other kinds of leadership research in that it normatively aims – directly or indirectly – at improving person-centred healthcare practice. Such research may be directed towards different levels of the healthcare system, be conducted within and across different scholarly disciplines, supported by different theories, and the use of different methods. We therefore propose a hybrid theoretical framework that aims at capturing a complex whole, putting the service user as person at the centre of attention, as illustrated in Figure 8.5.

REFERENCES

van den Akker, J., Gravemeijer, K., McKenney, S. and Nieveen, N. (eds) (2006) *Educational Design Research*. Routledge, London.

Alvesson, M. and Sköldberg, K. (2009) *Reflexive Methodology: New Vistas For Qualitative Research*, 2nd edition. Sage, London.

Bass, B. (1990) From transactional to transformational leadership: learning to share the vision. *Organizational Dynamics*, **8**, 19–31.

Beckett, P., Field, J., Molloy, L. *et al.* (2013) Practice what you preach: developing person-centred culture in inpatient mental health settings through strengths-based, transformational leadership. *Issues in Mental Health Nursing*, **34**, 595–601.

Bergold, J. and Thomas, S. (2012) Participatory research methods: a methodological approach in motion. *Forum: Qualitative Social Research*, **13**, Art. 30.

Binns, J. (2008) The ethics of relational leading: gender matters. *Gender, Work & Organization*, **15**, 600–620.

Boog, B. (2008) Afterthoughts: the ethos, epistemology and heuristics of participatory action research, in *Towards Quality Improvement of Action Research* (eds B. Boog, J. Preece, M. Slagter and J. Zeelen). Sense Publishers, Rotterdam. pp. 211–229.

Brooker, D. (2004) What is Person Centred Care for people with dementia? *Reviews in Clinical Gerontology*, **13**, 215–222.

Brooker, D. (2006) *Person-Centred Dementia Care Making Services Better*. Bradford Dementia Group Good Practice Guides. 160 pp.

Brown, M.E. and Treviño, L.K. (2003) Is values-based leadership ethical leadership?, in *Emerging perspectives on values in organizations* (eds S.W. Gilliand, D.D. Steiner and D.P. Skarlicki). Information Age Publishing, Greenwich. pp. 151–173.

Buber, M. (1923/37) *I and Thou* (trans. by Ronald Gregor Smith). T. & T. Clark, Edinburgh.

Cardiff, S. (2012) Critical and creative reflective inquiry: surfacing narratives to enable learning and inform action. *Educational Action Research*, **20**, 605–622.

Cardiff, S. (2014) *Person-Centred Leadership: A Critical Participatory Action Research Study Exploring and Developing a New Style of (Clinical) Nurse Leadership*. PhD Thesis. University of Ulster.

Cunliffe, A.L. and Eriksen, M. (2011) Relational leadership. *Human Relations*, **64**, 1425–1449.

Eide, T. (2010) Ibsen, leadership and morality. On Henrik Ibsen's *The Pretenders*, in *Heroes and Anti-heroes: European Literature and the Ethics of Leadership* (eds R. Ghesquière and K.J. Ims). Garant, Antwerpen. pp. 115–135.

Eide, T. and Aadland, E. (2012) *Etikkhåndboka for kommunenes helse- og omsorgstjenester [The ethics handbook for the municipalities' health and care services]*, 2nd edition. Kommuneforlaget, Oslo.

Eide, T., Bakken, L., Fauskanger, E.A. and Eide, H. (2014) *The Dream Project: Improving Organizational Communication in Primary Healthcare*. Paper presented at the 12th EACH International Conference on Communication in Health Care, Amsterdam.

Eide, T., van Dulmen, S. and Eide, H. (2016) Educating for ethical leadership through web-based coaching. a feasibility study. *Nursing Ethics*, **23**, 851–865.

Eide, T., Landmark, B. and Martinsen, T. (2015) *Refleksjonshåndboka for etisk lederskap i helse- og omsorgstjenestene [The ethical leadership reflection handbook for the health and care services]*. KS, Oslo.

Emery, M. and Purser, R. (1996) *The Search Conference: A Powerful Method for Planning Organizational Change and Community Action*. Jossey-Bass, San Francisco.

ENDA (2011) The European nurse directors' proto-code of ethics and conduct. http://www.enda-europe.com/en/publications.html (accessed 1 February 2017) *European Nurse Directors Association*.

Fay, B. (1987) *Critical Social Science: Liberation and its Limits*. Cornell University Press, New York.

Freire, P. (1970) *Pedagogy of the Oppressed*. Herder and Herder, New York.

Gillespie, A., Reader, T.W., Cornish, F. and Campbell, C. (2014) Beyond ideal speech situations: adapting to communication asymmetries in healthcare. *Journal of Health Psychology*, **19**, 72–78.

Gjerberg, E., Lillemoen, L., Dreyer, A., Pedersen, R. and Førde, R. (2014) Etisk kompetanseheving i norske kommuner – hva er gjort, og hva har vært levedyktig over tid? *Etikk i praksis*, **8**, 31–49.

Grant, J., Nelson, G. and Mitchell, T. (2008) Negotiating the challenges of participatory action research: relationships, power, participation, change and credibility, in *The SAGE Handbook of Action Research: Participative Inquiry and Practice*, 2nd edition (eds P. Reason and H. Bradbury). Sage, London. pp. 589–601.

Grill, C., Ahlborg, G. and Lindgren, E.C. (2011) Valuation and handling of dialogue in leadership; a grounded theory study in Swedish hospitals. *Journal of Health Organization and Management*, **25**, 34–54.

Habermas, J. (1984) *The Theory of Communicative Action*. Beacon Press, Boston.

Hersey, P., Blanchard, K.H. and Johnson, D.E. (2001) *Management of Organizational Behavior: Leading Human Resources*, 8th edition. Prentice-Hall, New Jersey.

HF (2014) *Person-Centred Care Made Simple*. The Health Foundation, London.

HOD (2015) *Fremtidens primærhelsetjeneste – nærhet og helhet Meld. St. 26 (2014-2015)* Helse-og omsorgsdepartementet, Oslo.

HSE (2011) *The Health Promotion Strategic Framework - Main Report*. Health Service Executive - National Health Promotion Office.

Høie, B. (2014) *Pasientens helsetjeneste [The patient's health and care service]*, January 7, https://www.regjeringen.no/no/aktuelt/pasientens-helsetjeneste/id748854/(accessed 1 February 2017) [The Norwegian Government, press release]

ICN (2012) *The ICN Code of Ethics for Nurses*. International Council of Nurses, Geneva.

Jakimowicz, S. and Perry, L. (2015) A concept analysis of patient-centred nursing in the intensive care unit. *Journal of Advanced Nursing*, **71**, 1499–1517.

Kant, I. (1785/2001) Grounding for the metaphysics of morals, in *Classics of Moral and Political Theory*, 3rd edition (ed. M. L. Morgan). Hackett, Indianapolis. pp. 833–873.

Kidd, D.C. and Castano, E. (2013) Reading literary fiction improves theory of mind. *Science*, **342**, 377–380.

Klaver, K. and Baart, A. (2011) Attentiveness in care: towards a theoretical framework. *Nursing Ethics*, **18**, 686–693.

Levin, M. (2014) Search conference, in *The SAGE Encyclopedia of Action Research* (eds D. Coghlan and M. Brydon-Miller). Jossey-Bass, San Francisco. pp. 696–699.

Liker, J.K. and Convis, G.L. (2012) *The Toyota Way to Lean Leadership – Achieving and Sustaining Excellence Through Leadership Development*. McGraw-Hill, New York.

Lynch, B.M., McCormack, B. and McCance, T. (2011) Development of a model of situational leadership in residential care for older people. *Journal of Nursing Management*, **19**, 1058–1069.

McCance, T., McCormack, B. and Dewing, J. (2011) An exploration of person-centredness in practice. *The Online Journal of Issues in Nursing*, **16**, Manuscript 1.

McConnell, D., McCance, T. and Melby, V. (2015) Exploring person-centredness in emergency departments: a literature review. *International Emergency Nursing*, **26**, 38–46.

McCormack, B. (2003) A conceptual framework for person-centred practice with older people. *International Journal of Nursing Practice*, **9**, 202–209.

McCormack, B. and McCance, T. (2010) *Person-Centred Nursing: Theory And Practice*. Wiley Blackwell, Oxford.

Manthey, M. (2009) The 40th anniversary of primary nursing: setting the record straight. *Creative Nursing*, **15**, 36–37.

Mead, N. and Bower, B. (2000) *Patient-centredness: a conceptual framework and review of the empirical literature*. Social Science and Medicine, **51**, 1087–1110.

Merriam, S. (1996) Updating our knowledge of adult learning. *The Journal of Continuing Education in the Health Professions*, **16**, 136–143.

Molven, O. and Ferkis, J. (eds) (2011) *Healthcare, Welfare and Law. Health Legislation as a Mirror of the Norwegian Welfare State*. Gyldendal Akademisk, Oslo.

NBHS (2013) *Annual Supervision Report 2012*. Norwegian Board of Health Supervision, Oslo.

NMHCS (2009) *The Coordination Reform. Proper Treatment – At The Right Place And Right Time. Report No. 47 (2008-2009) to the Storting*. Norwegian Ministry of Health and Care Services, Oslo.

Guarantee of Dignity (2010) *Forskrift om en verdig eldreomsorg (verdighetsgarantien) [Regulations on Dignified Elderly Care ('Guarantee of Dignity')]*. Retrieved from https://lovdata.no/dokument/SF/forskrift/2010-11-12-1426 (accessed 1 February 2017).

NMHCS (2013) *Future Care. Meld. St. 29 (2012–2013) Report to the Storting (white paper)*. Norwegian Ministry of Health and Care Services, Oslo.

NMHCS (2015) *The Primary Health and Care Services of Tomorrow – Localised and Integrated. Meld. St. 26 (2014–2015). Report to the Storting (white paper)*. Norwegian Ministry of Health and Care Services, Oslo.

Reason, P. and Bradbury, H. (2008) *The SAGE Handbook of Action Research. Participative Inquiry and Practice*, 2nd edition. Sage, London.

Ries, E. (2011) *The Lean Startup*. Crown Publishing, New York.

Rogers, C.R. (1961) *On Becoming a Person: A Therapist's View of Psychotherapy*. Houghton Mifflin, Boston.

Rokstad, A.M.M., Vatne, S., Engedal, K. and Selbaek, G. (2015) The role of leadership in the implementation of person-centred care using Dementia Care Mapping: a study in three nursing homes. *Journal of Nursing Management*, **23**, 15–26.

Scouller, J. (2011) *The Three Levels of Leadership: How to Develop Your Leadership Presence, Knowhow and Skill*. Management Books, Cirencester.

Senge, P.M., Scharmer, C.O., Jaworski, J. and Flowers, B.S. (2005) *Presence: Human Purpose and the Field of the Future*. Doubleday, New York.

Snoeren, M. (2015) *Working = Learning. A Complexity Approach to Workplace Learning within Residential Care for Older People*. PhD Thesis, VU University Medical Centre Amsterdam, Ridderkerk.

Söderhamn, U., Kjøstvedt, H.T. and Slettebø, Å. (2014) Evaluation of ethical reflections in community healthcare: a mixed-methods study. *Nursing Ethics*, **22**, 194–204.

Steiger, N.J. and Balog, A. (2010) Realizing patient-centered care: putting patients in the center, not the middle. *Frontiers of Health Services Management*, **26**, 15–25.

Storch, J., Makaroff, K.S., Pauly, B. and Newton, L. (2013) Take me to my leader: the importance of ethical leadership among formal nurse leaders. *Nursing Ethics*, **20**, 150–157.

Uhl-Bien, M. (2006) Relational leadership theory: exploring the social processes of leadership and organizing. *The Leadership Quarterly*, **17**, 654–676.

Winter, R. and Munn-Giddings, C. (eds) (2001) *A Handbook for Action Research in Health and Social Care*. Routledge, London.

World Health Organization (2009) *Milestones in Health Promotion*. World Health Organization, Geneva.

Introduction to Section 2

DOING PERSON-CENTRED RESEARCH: METHODS IN ACTION

This section of the book brings to life the philosophical, theoretical and methodological perspectives discussed in Section 1. The researchers and academics leading these chapters are engaged in person-centred research and are every day, grappling with the challenges of doing research in a person-centred way.

The chapters will aim to present:

- An overview of a study or area of research if not based on a single research project.
- Principles of person-centredness guiding the study/research area.
- Process and outcome evaluation used.
- Study progress and/or key findings/impacts on persons, people, populations.
- Reflections on doing person-centred research and being a person-centred researcher.
- Key learning.

Each chapter includes reflective questions at the beginning, to be considered when reading the chapter. Each chapter will end with a short commentary by the Editors of the book. This commentary will challenge, critique and appraise the perspectives offered and engage the reader in a critical discussion of the chapter and issues raised. Consideration of the reflective questions posed at the beginning of the chapter will enable the reader to engage with the Editors' Commentary.

Person-Centred Healthcare Research, First Edition. Edited by Brendan McCormack, Sandra van Dulmen, Hilde Eide, Kirsti Skovdahl and Tom Eide.
© 2017 John Wiley & Sons Ltd. Published 2017 by John Wiley & Sons Ltd.

9 Staffing Structures for Effectiveness in Person-Centred Care: The RAFAELA® System

Lisbeth Fagerström

Reflective questions

1. What are the theoretical foundations of the RAFAELA® system?
2. What are the motivations and rationale for monitoring daily patients' individual care needs and nurses' workload?
3. How can the nurse manager, by using the data of the RAFAELA® system, promote person-centred care?

INTRODUCTION

The RAFAELA® system was developed in Finland in the mid-1990s. As a result of the banking crisis that ravaged the country at the time, the Finnish healthcare system was subject to substantial budgetary cuts and demands for fiscal austerity. Unfortunately, the economic situation we are facing today both domestically in Finland and throughout Europe is similar to the 1990s. Our healthcare systems today are under great pressure from cost savings and so-called 'efficiency improvements'. The fact remains that salaries are one of the largest expenditures within most healthcare systems and, just like in the 1990s, the budget for care staff salaries will most likely be subject to significant austerity requirements. The combination of over-indebted countries together with ageing populations may result in economically difficult times for most European countries' healthcare systems.

In this delicate balancing act – where quality should be continuously improved alongside a major focus on patient (service user) safety, where service user demands are increasing yet economic resources are ever more limited – new methods and systems are needed whereby these factors can be monitored and managed. International research has demonstrated that nursing resources, in terms of both educational levels and number of nurses, are clearly linked to quality indicators, patient safety, results and mortality (Aiken *et al.*, 2010, 2014). An effective and balanced allocation of personnel resources will therefore promote person-centred care for patients.

The question is not only about increasing staff resources, but is also about how available resources can be allocated in the best possible manner and how service users can be guaranteed high quality, safe and person-centred care. New methods are needed for leaders and healthcare administrators to develop and guarantee person-centred care for patients.

Person-Centred Healthcare Research, First Edition. Edited by Brendan McCormack, Sandra van Dulmen, Hilde Eide, Kirsti Skovdahl and Tom Eide.
© 2017 John Wiley & Sons Ltd. Published 2017 by John Wiley & Sons Ltd.

OVERVIEW OF THE RAFAELA® SYSTEM

The RAFAELA® system was developed for hospital settings in Finland in the late 1990s. Using this scientifically tested tool, a nurse manager is able to balance service users' care needs and nursing resources so as to create an optimal nurse staffing level. The main idea is that the workload per nurse (expressed in NI points per nurse) should be on the optimal NI level, and thereby assure the quality of nursing, patient outcomes, good working conditions for staff and an effective use of available resources. The validity of the RAFAELA® system's measurement tools and the system's feasibility for human resource management in nursing has been assessed in several studies, including four PhD theses (Fagerström, 1999; Pusa, 2007; Rauhala, 2008; Frilund, 2013).

The RAFAELA® system has been developed based on a person-centred perspective, where each individual's care needs constitute the starting point for care and a clear focus is placed on the work situation for care staff and nursing intensity (NI; Fagerström, Lønning and Andersen, 2014) The driving force behind the development of the RAFAELA® system has been and still is the promotion of fundamental care tasks, such as guaranteeing good and safe care and contributing to 'making good care possible'.

The development of a system for the classification and measurement of NI started in the 1940s in the USA. In the 1980s the number of systems and instruments began to noticeably increase. Prior to the introduction and general use of computers, the use and benefits of collecting large amounts of data were limited (Fagerström, 1999). Information technology has enabled the collection of data and eased the compiling of reports, allowing for a more effective manner of assessing and managing data than previously. Today, we can ask why do we really need a system for systematic classification and daily measurement of service users' care needs, the nursing intensity and the nurses' workload? Based on previous research and literature, there are three main motivations:

1. Guarantee care along with quality standards and good care outcomes.
2. Guarantee an optimal allocation and calculation of staff resources.
3. Promote and develop evidence-based leadership.

By means of daily and systematic use of the RAFAELA® system, the managers and leaders on different levels of the organisation can get a comprehensive picture of care needs and a realistic picture of the needs for nurse staffing resources, which is assessed as an important aspect of progressive management. Systematic use of the data provides the possibility for local, regional and national comparisons (benchmarking). Benchmarking can lead to 'benchlearning', which means that we can learn from other organisations where leaders and organisations have succeed in creating good working conditions that promote person-centred care (Fagerström and Rauhala, 2007).

THE THEORETICAL FOUNDATIONS OF THE RAFAELA® SYSTEM

The RAFAELA® system is based on a holistic view of persons from a caring and nursing science perspective. In addition it recognises nursing as being comprised of complex caring components (Fagerström, 2000, 2009). The holistic view of the person is a central ontological starting point. To understand the unique service user and the person that he/she is while taking into account his/her actual life context cannot be emphasised enough. Each person should be helped to experience that his/her physical, social and spiritual/existential needs are noted and addressed. The service user should be in the centre of all healthcare services (McCormack and McCance, 2010), and the working conditions for nurses are an important pre-requisite for person-centred nursing. The humanitarian view of the human being is also a starting point for the development of both the Oulu Patient Classification (OPCq) instrument and the PAONCIL (Professional Assessment of Optimal Nursing Care Intensity Level) method (Fagerström *et al.*, 2000a), which are parts of the RAFAELA® system. The OPCq instrument consists of both physical and mental health needs and the nursing activities related to these. Included in the OPCq instrument are conversations with and emotional support for service users and their relatives, which can be considered unique to classification systems of this type.

The PAONCIL method is based on an assessment of actual care needs and the work situation of the staff. According to Human Resource Management, the persons/the staff in an organisation are the most central resource and it is the staff that can 'make a difference' for the users (Storey, 1989). The PAONCIL method is defined as a 'bottom-up' method for the allocation of staff resources, which is in accordance also with the person-centred perspective. The allocation of resources emanating from a 'top-down' leadership style is not compatible with the RAFAELA® system. The PAONCIL method builds on trust between the nurse leader and the staff. The allocation of resources should derive from service users' care needs, and it is only the nurses who 'know the person' who can determine these needs. The nurse that knows the service user as a person is able to assess his/her needs, wishes and worries. As the nurse has to know the service user, the nurse leader has to know the nurses' work situation.

Staff should not be perceived merely in terms of costs, which should be reduced by all means possible, but instead as a resource for care and essential to the realisation of necessary goals (Storey, 1989). Staff as a resource and a 'competitive factor', and their competence level is of crucial importance for person-centred care (McCormack and McCance, 2010). It is of great importance to the end result of the care provided, that staff commit to the activities, in this case primarily in regard to service users, that they are asked to engage in. In Human Resource Management, work conditions and the work environment as well as the competence level of the staff are important for good results (Vuori, 2005). Leaders' commitment is crucial for the outcomes and nurse managers should take full responsibility for the planning of staff and other resources. If care leaders do not take responsibility and engage themselves in the nurses' work situation and workload, the allocation of resources and the management of care activities, the daily and systematic classification of patients will also not be successful. When nurse managers are interested in systematic follow-up and monitoring of their staff's workload, this is concrete evidence for engagement, caring for and interest in their staff's well-being, comfort and work satisfaction. Consequently, their effort will promote person-centred care.

DEFINITION OF CENTRAL CONCEPTS

The concept of 'nursing intensity' is closely related to the concepts 'patient dependency', 'acuity' and 'severity'. The use of such concepts implies that intensity relates to how nursing intensive (demanding) a situation is and how dependent a service user is on the care provided, that is to say how much care, help and support a service user receives when in care, during a certain period of time (usually 24 hours; Fagerström, 1999).

The concept of 'intensity' should not be considered equivalent to the concept of 'workload'. 'Workload', and a nurse's total workload, includes more than the 'mere' effort exerted and the nursing activities that stem from meeting care needs. The total nursing workload is defined as the sum of direct and indirect patient-related nursing activities, non-patient nursing activities and central non-patient factors: those staff/nurse-related, contextual and/or organisational factors that may affect nurses' experiences of their total workload (Fagerström and Vainikainen, 2014).

COMPONENTS OF THE RAFAELA® SYSTEM

By means of the scientifically tested RAFAELA® system, a nurse manager is able to balance patients' care needs and the nursing resources needed to fulfil these needs in a manner that equates to optimal nurse staffing (Fagerström, 1999; Rauhala, 2008; Fagerström *et al.*, 2014).

The RAFAELA® system currently consists of the following components (see Figure 9.1):

1. *Instruments for measuring NI in different contexts*: daily registration of service users by the OPCq – a generic instrument for all specialties in hospital; PPCq for mental health care; POLIHOIq for outpatient units and emergency services, PERIHOIq for operating and recovery rooms, day-surgery; SÄDEHOIq for radiation therapy.
2. *Staff resources:* daily registration of actual nursing staff resources (in numbers, on 0.25 level).
3. *Determination of optimal NI level*: by means of the PAONCIL instrument during a period of 4–6 weeks.
4. *Financial information:* participating organisations send additional information to a national centre annually, including financial information for calculation of costs and benchmarking purposes.

The validity of the Oulu Patient Classification instrument (OPCq), developed for a hospital setting, has been tested from different perspectives (expert panels, service users, both qualitatively and quantitatively) in Finland and Norway (Fagerström, Bergbom and Eriksson, 1998; Fagerström 2000; Fagerström and Rauhala 2003; Frilund and Fagerström, 2009; Andersen, Lønning and Fagerström, 2014). The reliability of the OPCq should be tested annually by parallel classifications at each unit where the system is in daily use. The OPCq

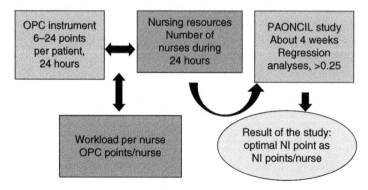

Figure 9.1   The components of the RAFAELA® system. Source: Courtesy of L. Fagerström.

instrument, developed for a hospital setting, is used to measure service users' daily (in the afternoon; 24 hours retrospectively) NI. The OPCq instrument consists of the following six subareas of needs and nursing activities:

1. Planning and co-ordination of nursing care.
2. Breathing, blood circulation and symptoms of disease.
3. Nutrition and medication.
4. Personal hygiene and secretion.
5. Activity, sleep and rest.
6. Teaching, guidance in care and follow-up care, emotional support (Fagerström, 1999).

The NI for each subarea can vary from 1 to 4 points. The points are added up, giving a range of 6–24 NI points per person (see Figure 9.2). The total sum of NI points for all service users in the unit is then calculated, for example 280 points. Then the total sum of NI points for a unit is divided by the total number of nurses who had worked on the unit during that calendar day. Giving an example of 10 nurses, the actual workload per nurse would then be, in this case, 28 NI points per nurse. The first version of the OPCq was developed for use in specialist healthcare. During the past few years, new versions suitable to different contexts, such as POLIHOIq for outpatient units and emergency services, the PPC (Pitkäniemi Patient Classification) for mental healthcare services, the PERIHOIq version for operating and recovery rooms and day-surgery, and SÄDEHOIq for radiation therapy units.

The implementation process of the RAFAELA® system takes about 6 months. After the implementation and testing the reliability of the OPCq classifications, the *Professional Assessment of Optimal Care Intensity Level* (PAONCIL) study can begin. The PAONCIL method is an alternative to classical time studies and can be described as *nurses' professional assessment of the sufficiency of resources in relation to the actual NI of patients during a*

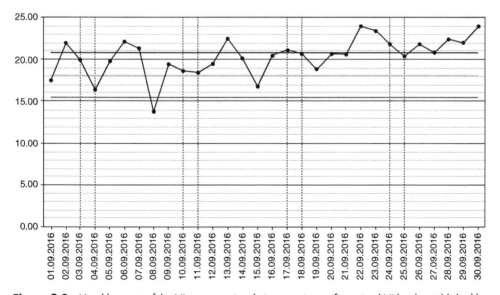

Figure 9.2 Monthly report of the NI per nurse in relation to unit specific optimal NI level, established by means of the PAONCIL method, July 2011 on a surgical unit in Finland. Source: National Benchmarking Report, Finnish Consulting Group Ltd; http://www.rafaela.fi/?q=en.

shift (Fagerström *et al.*, 2000b; Rauhala and Fagerström, 2004, 2007). The validity and credibility of the PAONCIL method, including the manual, has been evaluated in several studies (Fagerström and Rainio, 1999; Fagerström *et al.*, 2000b; Fagerström, Nojonen and Åkers, 2002; Fagerström and Vainikainen, 2014).

Optimal NI is defined as the intensity that every trained professional nurse working in the unit can handle without compromising the standard of good nursing care determined for the unit. The level of optimal NI may vary by 15% to either side of the optimal point. This creates an optimal area (see Figure 9.2) for NI, similar to a 'good reference point' for the unit, and the goal is that the workload per nurse should be on this optimal level most of the days: for example 70% of days.

Using the PAONCIL method, an optimal NI level is determined for each unit on the basis of nurses' professional assessments during a period of time lasting at least 3–4 weeks. Each nurse makes an overall assessment at the end of each shift or before leaving the unit, determining whether the nursing resources have been sufficient in relation to patients' needs and NI, using a scale from –3 to +3. A PAONCIL score of zero (0) is considered optimal and indicates that the number of nurses is balanced with patients' needs and NI and that nurses have a realistic opportunity to provide good care. The optimal staffing level of a unit can be established through the linear regression analysis of the results of the OPCq points per nurse and PAONCIL scores. The PAONCIL instrument also includes additional questions that can reveal non-patient factors (other than NI) that may increase or decrease nurses' workload during a specific work shift. By analysing these non-patient factors, the nurse manager gains an idea of which other factors (organising and planning of work, manager's role, staff situation, meetings, training events and other absences, students, cooperation with doctors, etc.) may be either stressing care staff or easing the overall work situation (Rauhala and Fagerström, 2007).

THE BENEFITS OF THE SYSTEMATIC AND DAILY USE OF THE RAFAELA® SYSTEM

The RAFAELA® system is above all a management tool that can be integrated into an organisation's overall leadership, management and patient administrative system. It builds on actual data on service users' care needs and nurses' workload and provides an efficient platform for the management of nursing resources, both operatively and strategically. However, the system has also a clear impact on nurses' clinical practice and thereby affects patient outcomes. With the help of the RAFAELA® system nursing management and leadership become more effective. Among other things the system makes it possible to:

1. *Improve person-centred care*: every service user is unique and their needs vary over time. Daily monitoring/classifying of their actual care needs constitutes a clear structure of nursing care and promotes a person-centred approach.
2. *Improve quality and manage risks better*: real care needs (not just the number of service users or their diagnoses) are taken into account and optimal workload per nurse reduces mistakes and adverse events and improves patient safety.
3. *Improve workforce planning and decrease staff costs*: savings come from (for example) the effective allocation of available resources, including the decreased need for deputy nurses, acute replacements or permanent reserves. Provides information for cost accounting and budgetary decisions.

4. *Increase nurses' job satisfaction and decrease sick-leave*: Resources are allocated in an optimal manner, which results in a more well balanced and more equally distributed workload.
5. *Enhance the quality of documented care*: Nurses' daily and systematic classifications by the OPCq are based on both the nurses' own experiences and the nursing documentation. Better documentation gives a more reliable classification of patients' NI.

The RAFAELA® system provides a variety of information that can be used for different purposes by staff nurses, nurse managers on different levels, top-level managers and politicians. Below are some examples of *how a nurse manager can apply the information in her/ his leadership when developing care quality and person-centred care and in evidence-based human resource management.*

Professional and high quality nursing starts from the individual service user and his/her care needs. For example, those experiencing an infarct of the brain (DRG 14; for example 17 NI points/day) have on average a higher NI than service users with rhythmic cardiac disease (DRG 139; 13 NI points/day). When comparing the two types of service user, some factors should be taken into account. For example, the average age of a person with a cardiac infarct is lower and, generally, such people can take care of their own personal hygiene. A brain infarct often leads to aphasia, decreased physical functioning and the need for guidance in self-care at discharge and follow-up care. There are two clear advantages of the OPCq not common to other instruments for measuring NI:

1. The OPCq's first needs subarea (planning and coordination of care) and sixth needs subarea (teaching, guidance in care and follow-up care, emotional support; also includes relatives' need for support and guidance). It has proven to be a wise decision to include the first needs subarea (planning and coordination of care) in the system, despite that this domain has traditionally been grouped under indirect care.
2. Today, effectively planned care is one condition for efficient care pathways. The value and importance of person-centred health information, mentoring, trust and support cannot be underestimated in nursing. For example, children living with diabetes and their parents need support and guidance in self-care during the hospital stay. Critics may assess the OPCq instrument as being rather 'broad' with only six needs subareas, but when classification of each person's care needs and NI occurs daily, the data provides a sensitive picture of service users' constantly changing acuity. The structure of the OPCq reminds nurses what the most central nursing dimensions are. The nurse manager can use reports about NI during a discussion about care quality: referring to the use of working time, the prioritisation of nursing activities, etc. Nurse managers typically hold monthly meetings with their staff and discuss NI profiles and even hold such discussions at the clinical level with the management team.

In Figure 9.2 we see an example of the main idea with the RAFAELA® system that is nurses' actual workload in relation to the optimal NI level of a unit as measured using the PAONCIL instrument. When the RAFAELA® system is in daily use, the nurse manager can plan and reallocate staff proactively on the basis of the last day and/or the last period, allowing him/her to adjust the staffing level so that optimal workload is achieved. Such resource allocation can even be applied between units and clinics. On the specific unit seen in Figure 9.2, the nurses' workload has been on the optimal NI level for 58% of the days (18 days) while care needs were higher than staff resources for 23% of the days. We also see that the nurses experienced six 'easy' days with low workload. This report clearly shows whether the average workload per nurse has increased, decreased or remained at the same level, and these reports can consist of per-monthly data or data from several years, helping for example to discern seasonal trends. This allows a Director of Nursing or an Executive to compare the workload per nurse between units and/or clinics and even between hospitals, which is possible if several hospitals are using the RAFAELA® system.

According to nurse managers, these reports are especially useful when discussing the need for the reallocation of staff and for the future planning of staff resources. An interesting question is whether, for example, it is possible to reorganise a unit's activities in order to yield a more stable workload per nurse, on the optimal NI level. After organisational changes or extensive staff changes a new PAONCIL study should be undertaken, and the recommendation is that this occurs every second or third year for normal situations. Such reports are easy to understand for managers on different levels in the organisation and for politicians. Also service users and their relatives may benefit from an understandable picture of the situation on the unit; perhaps the person will choose this unit again in the future having seen the nurses' work situation. Still, if 50% of days are over the optimal NI level, would the person choose this unit/hospital again in the future? Already today in some countries, service users have the right to choose which hospital they receive care from.

In Figure 9.3 we see a benchmarking report that shows days, in percentages, above the optimal NI level (red areas), on the optimal NI level (green areas), and under the optimal NI level (yellow areas). Such reporting builds on the idea of the 'traffic light' reporting system, where one bar can represent one unit, clinic/division, hospital, region or country. This is a benchmarking report from Finland and shows the workload situation of the nurses at one hospital in 2011 (16 units). As a

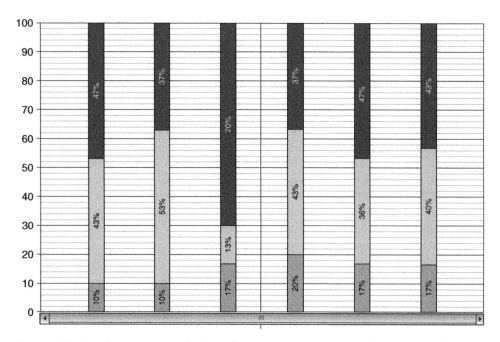

Figure 9.3 Sample, comparative database from RAFAELA®. The optimal NI level on 16 units in Finland, 2011. Source: National Benchmarking Report, Finnish Consulting Group Ltd; http://rafaela.fi/ sites/default/files/Rafaela/Public/BIT_Rafaela_hoitoisuusluokitusj%C3%A4rjestelm%C3% A4_ENGLISH_web.pdf.

Nurse Executive, Director of Nursing or Coordinator of nursing staff a descriptive overall picture of the nurses' workload can be obtained. This can be compared to other kinds of reports, for example pertaining to job satisfaction, sick-leave, adverse events, nurse-to-patient ratios, etc.

CONCLUSIONS AND REFLECTIONS ON BEING A PERSON-CENTRED NURSE LEADER WHEN DEALING WITH NURSE STAFFING ISSUES

After more than 15 years of experience of the RAFAELA® system it is possible to conclude that a systematic registration of staff resources and the classification of NI increases care leaders' consciousness of the relationship between care needs and resources. A longitudinal study also highlighted this tendency, in other words that the systematic use of the RAFAELA® system increases awareness of the allocation of resources and that as a result an organisation's leadership becomes more aware and goal-oriented in their actions (Fagerström, 2009). The strengths of the RAFAELA® system include:

- its classification system is person-centred;
- it is not time consuming and it is not difficult for users to learn how to use;
- continuous reliability testing ensures reliable data;
- it has been validated in Finland and Norway; and
- it is relatively easy to compile and use reports generated by the system.

The systematic use of the system and participation in national benchmarking provides opportunities for nation-to-nation comparisons. However, for the time being this possibility is perhaps not fully utilised by those organisations that employ the system. One weakness is that not all patient record systems have yet been made electronic, which would facilitate easy electronic classification. A further weakness is the fact that, at present, the competence level of staff and its importance to the allocation of staff resources is not currently included in the system. This should be considered in the further development of the system. However, a comparable and scientifically tested classification system whereby NI can be measured does not currently exist in Europe.

The RAFAELA® system is based on scientific research, and nurses and managers feel that it is an easy but, at the same time, a somewhat complex system to use. According to our experiences, the implementation process is rather resource/time consuming. Nevertheless, the implementation process is also a learning process for both nurses and leaders on different levels and helps initiate discussions about 'what is good nursing care?' and 'are there realistic work conditions for person-centred nursing?' along all processes. In Kane and colleagues' systematic review and meta-analyses (Kane *et al.*, 2007), an association between RN staffing (nurse–patient ratios) and lower odds of hospital-related mortality and adverse patient events was found. In their discussion of the results they point out that the strength of the association between nurse staffing and patient outcomes can be affected by the method whereby staff resources are calculated. The foundation of the RAFAELA® system is that of service user care needs and NI, not nurse–patient ratios. According to Lang *et al.* (2004), the literature offers minimal support for specific minimum nurse–patient ratios for units in acute care hospitals, and a minimum nurse–patient ratio alone seems to be inadequate in ensuring quality of care. They recommend that service user acuity, skill mix, nurse competence, and other central variables should be considered when realising staffing requirements.

KEY LEARNING

The systematic use of the RAFAELA® system provides care leaders with reliable data that can be used for evidence-based leadership. The allocation of staff resources should emanate from service user care needs and NI. If this occurs, then a fundamental condition for the guaranteeing of good care for service users is fulfilled.

REFERENCES

Aiken, L.H., Sloane, D.M., Ciniotti, J.P. *et al.* (2010) Implications of the California nurse staffing mandate for other states. *Health Services Research*, **45**, 904–921.

Aiken, L.H., Sloane, D.M., Bruyneel, L. *et al.* (2014) Nurse staffing and education and hospital mortality in nine European countries: a retrospective observational study. *Lancet*, **383**, 1824–1830.

Andersen, M.H., Lønning, K. and Fagerström, L. (2014) Testing reliability and validity of the Oulu Patient Classification Instrument—the first step in evaluating the RAFAELA System in Norway. *Open Journal of Nursing*, **4**, 303–311. Published Online April 2014 in SciRes. http://dx.doi.org/10.4236/ojn.2014.44035 (accessed 1 February 2017).

Fagerström, L. (1999) *The Patient's Caring Needs. To Understand and Measure the Unmeasurable*. Doctoral Thesis, Åbo Akademi University, Åbo, Finland.

Fagerström, L. (2000) Expertvalidering av Oulu Patient Classification - en fas i utvecklingen av ett nytt system för vårdtyngdsklassificering, RAFAELA. [*Expert evaluation of the Oulu Patient Classification - a phase in the development of a new system of patient classification, RAFAELA*]. *Nordic Journal of Nursing Science*, **20**, 15–21.

Fagerström, L. (2009) Evidence-based human resource management: a study of nurse leaders' resource allocation. *Journal of Nursing Management*, **17**, 415–425.

Fagerström, L., Bergbom, I. E. and Eriksson, E. (1998) A comparison between patients' experience of how their caring needs have been met and the nurses' patient classification - an explorative study. *Journal of Nursing Management*, **6**, 978–987.

Fagerström, L., Lønning, K. and Andersen, M.H. (2014) The RAFAELA system: a workforce planning tool for nurse staffing and human resource management. *Nursing Management*, **21**, 30–36.

Fagerström, L., Nojonen, K. and Åkers, A. (2002) Metodologinen triangulaatio Paoncil- menetelmän sisällön validiteetin testaamisessa. [*Methodological triangulation as a validation method in the testing of the PAONCIL method*]. *Journal of Nursing Science*, **14**, 180–191.

Fagerström, L. and Rainio, A-K. (1999) Professional assessment of optimal nursing care intensity – a new method for assessment of staffing levels for nursing care. *Journal of Clinical Nursing*, **8**, 369–379.

Fagerström, L., Rainio, A-K., Rauhala, A. and Nojonen, K. (2000a) Validation of a new method for patient classification, the Oulu Patient Classification. *Journal of Advanced Nursing*, **31**, 481–490.

Fagerström, L., Rainio, A-K., Rauhala, A. and Nojonen, K. (2000b) Professional assessment of optimal nursing care intensity level a new method for resource allocation as an alternative to classical time studies. *Scandinavian Journal of Caring Sciences*, **14**, 97–104.

Fagerström, L. and Rauhala, A. (2003) Finnhoitoisuus – hoitotyön benchmarking Projektin loppuraportti [*Finn Nursing Intensity–nursing workload benchmarking, Final project report*]. 2000–2002, SuomenKuntaliitto, Helsinki.

Fagerström, L. and Rauhala, A. (2007) Benchmarking in nursing care by the RAFAELA patient classification system. *Journal of Nursing Management*, **15**, 683–692.

Fagerström, L. and Vainikainen, P. (2014) Nurses' experiences of non-patient factors that affect nursing workload – a study of the PAONCIL instrument's non-patient factors. *Nursing Research and Practice* 2014:167674.

Frilund, M. (2013) *A Synthesiser of Caritative Ethics and Nursing Intensity*. Doctoral Thesis (in Swedish), Åbo Akademi University, Åbo, Finland.

Frilund, M. and Fagerström, L. (2009) Validity and reliability testing of the Oulu patient classification: instrument within primary health care for the older people. *International Journal of Older People Nursing*, **4**, 280–287.

Kane, R.L., Shamliyan, T.A., Mueller, C. *et al.* (2007) The association of registered nurse staffing levels and patient outcomes: systematic review and meta-analysis. *Medical Care*, **45**, 1195–1204.

Lang, T.A., Hodge, M., Olson, V. *et al.* (2004) Nurse-patient ratios: a systematic review on the effects of nurse staffing on patient, nurse employee, and hospital outcomes. *Journal of Nursing Administration*, **34**, 326–337.

McCormack, B. and McCance, T. (2010) *Person-Centred Nursing: Theory, Models and Methods.* Wiley Blackwell, Oxford.

Pusa, A-K. (2007) *The Right Nurse in the Right Place. Nursing Productivity and Utilisation of the RAFAELA Patient Classification System in Nursing Management.* Doctoral Thesis, University of Kuopio, Finland.

Rauhala, A. (2008) The Validity and Feasibility of Measurement Tools of Human Resources Management in Nursing. PhD Dissertation, Department of Health Policy and Management, University of Kuopio, Vaasa Central Hospital, Kuopio.

Rauhala, A. and Fagerström, L. (2004) Determining optimal nursing intensity: the RAFAELA method. *Journal of Advanced Nursing*, **45**, 351–359.

Rauhala, A. and Fagerström, L. (2007) Are nurses' assessments of their workload affected by non-patient factors? An analysis of the RAFAELA-system. *Journal of Nursing Management*, **15**, 490–499.

Storey, J. (1989) Introduction: from personnel management to human resource management, in *New Perspectives on Human Resource Management* (ed. J. Storey). Routledge, London.

Vuori, J. (ed.) (2005) Terveysjajohtaminen. Terveyshallintotiedeterveydenhuollontyöyhteisössä. [*Health and management. The science of healthcare management in cooperation with the healthcare system*]. WSOY, Helsinki.

Editors' Commentary

Determining the optimal nursing staff levels to provide the best possible care to service users and ensure patient safety and effective care outcomes is a key agenda in person-centred practice. Indeed, 'appropriate skill-mix' is one of the key prerequisites for person-centred practice in the person-centred practice framework of McCormack and McCance (2017). Research into nursing staffing levels and its relationship with quality care provision has been in progress for many years, with the 'holy grail' of the perfect workload allocation model still being sought. The recent pan-European research into nursing staffing (the RN4Cast study http://www.thelancet.com/journals/lancet/article/PIIS0140-6736(13)62631-8/abstract) produced the strongest evidence thus far of the relationship between adequate staffing and patient outcome. However, the research into nursing staffing models has largely been mechanistic in nature and has often been criticised for being reductionist and overly focused on objective measures of the observable tasks of nursing. Lisbeth Fagerström's research in this area of nursing work spans nearly 20 years of activity and the RAFAELA® system focuses on allocating the nursing resource according to the assessed care needs of service users. The system so far has only been used in Finland and Norway. Like many other systems RAFAELA® is connected with the acuity of care needs of service users, and whilst there is a 'simple' logic underpinning such a relationship, the reality of person-centred care provision is that it requires consideration of many other issues alongside acuity. The strength of RAFAELA® lies in the fact that it tries not to be reductionist by only focusing on six care domains rather than a long list of tasks/nursing inputs. However, as Fagerström herself acknowledges, nurse competency and expertise does not feature in the allocation formula. While it is true that few nursing-staffing allocation frameworks do consider competence and expertise, it seems that this is a critical area for further research. The RN4Cast study did correlate nursing expertise with patient morality (through a focus on the relationship between morality, staffing levels and the percentage of nurses who were graduates). Much more work is needed in this area to really understand the knowledge, skills and expertise of registered nurses in the context of a decision-making model such as RAFAELA®. From a person-centred perspective, it is not enough to focus on acuity alone as some of the most demanding (of nursing expertise) needs that service users may have are often when they are in a state of recovery and significant bio-psychosocial, cultural and personal care needs become the focus. In their person-centred practice framework, McCormack and McCance (2017) place skill mix alongside other prerequisites for effective person-centred practice, such as professional competence, interpersonal skills, beliefs and values, commitment to the job and knowing self. There is a need to determine the interrelationships between these prerequisites and how they impact on service user experience, care outcomes, as well as the overall quality of the person-centred culture in a nursing unit. Extending and further developing the RAFAELA® research in this direction may be a fruitful endeavour as well as engaging with other countries across Europe and beyond.

McCormack, B. and McCance, T. (2017) *Person-Centred Practice in Nursing and Healthcare: Theory and Practice*. Wiley Blackwell, Oxford.

10 Giving Voice to 'Hard To Reach Groups' in Healthcare Research: A Narrative Approach

Catherine Buckley

Reflective questions

1. How does an understanding of the values, beliefs, wants and wishes of older people enable therapeutic care to occur in residential care settings?
2. In what way does the implementation of a narrative approach to care and a focus on listening to the voices of older people enable nurses to operationalise person-centred care?
3. Does the use of a narrative approach enable the voice of older adults in residential care to be heard?

OVERVIEW OF THE STUDY

Narratives, life stories and stories have all been used in nursing research to explicate lives and value human experience (Frid, Ohlen and Bergbom, 2000). They can provide insight into how people cope with illness or how they experience their journey through the healthcare system. Narrative and biography give us an insight into what is unique about the person (Hardy, Gregory and Ramjett, 2009). Through capturing these stories and the meanings ascribed to them by individuals, researchers and practitioners can improve their understanding of the lived experience of the person and assist those in positions of vulnerability. Approximately 8% of the world's population is aged 65 or older. Similar to global trends, approximately 6% of older people in Ireland are receiving residential care. Personal identity and self-esteem are often not recognised in either services or support arrangements in particular for this vulnerable group. It is therefore particularly important that researchers give voice to this 'hard to reach group'. Narrative and the use of narrative in research and practice can help ensure that these voices are privileged in everyday care experiences and in the development of plans of care that put the person and their wishes, desires and wants first.

Person-Centred Healthcare Research, First Edition. Edited by Brendan McCormack, Sandra van Dulmen, Hilde Eide, Kirsti Skovdahl and Tom Eide.
© 2017 John Wiley & Sons Ltd. Published 2017 by John Wiley & Sons Ltd.

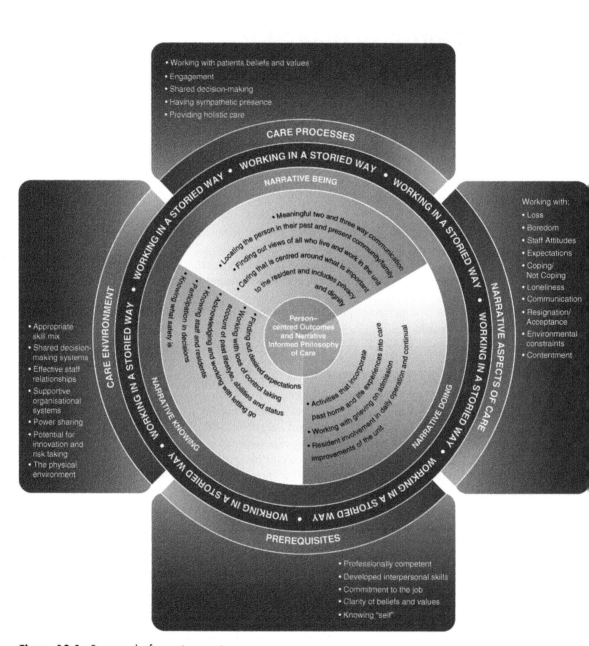

Figure 10.1 Framework of narrative practice.

This chapter will focus on the development, implementation and evaluation of a methodological framework for a narrative-based approach to practice development and person-centred care in residential aged care settings. Carried out between 2010 and 2014 and underpinned by theories of narrative inquiry, person-centred care, practice development and AR, the study is guided by the philosophical perspectives of Heidegger (1962). Forty-six interviews collected as part of a national research programme (Person-centred Practice Development Programme 2007–2010), were analysed for key themes by me and then through four focus groups with 12 clinical nurse managers and two independent experts. Themes were also derived from a focus group of eight residents who explored person-centredness and narrative. The combined analyses led to a single set of themes that was used to develop a Framework of Narrative Practice (Buckley, McCormack and Ryan, 2014) (Figure 10.1). This Framework consists of four pillars, prerequisites, care processes, care environment and narrative aspects of care. To operationalise the framework of narrative practice, three narrative elements – narrative knowing, narrative being and narrative doing, need to be considered. Working with the foundational pillars and the narrative elements enabled staff to 'work in a storied way' taking account of the voice of older people. Using the framework in practice allowed the stories and voices of this vulnerable group to inform their care and led to the development of person-centred outcomes and a narrative-informed philosophy of care.

The framework was implemented in practice, in two residential care settings (Unit 1 and Unit 2), comprising 37 residents and 38 staff, using an action research (AR) approach, with work-based learning groups. Three action cycles: (i) narrative practice and culture identification, (ii) developing narrative practice and (iii) working in a storied way emerged during the implementation. Using these action cycles, staff developed action plans to address areas where changes could improve practice and quality of life for the residents. These included communication/intercommunication, homely environment, having more going on with and for the residents, and meals and mealtimes.

The framework confirmed the identity and voices of older people by taking account of their biography. However, three key areas emerged that warranted further conceptualisation. These were: how staff and residents responded to change (narrative being), development of shared understandings (narrative knowing) and intentional action (narrative doing). It is these areas on which this chapter will focus.

PRINCIPLES OF PERSON-CENTREDNESS GUIDING THE STUDY

Central to the Person-Centred Nursing (PCN) framework (McCormack and McCance, 2010), is knowing the self and by extension knowing others. It involves knowing the values of the resident but also being clear about one's own values and beliefs. Similarly, narrative approaches promote a culture of caring because they value the voice, not only of the storyteller but also that of the listener/reteller (Bochner, 2001). Knowledge, i.e. narrative knowledge, can promote a more caring relationship where the narrative can influence the way care is carried out or planned. Narrative deals with meanings, contexts and perspectives and this is similar to the PCN framework that enables understanding. It privileges a person-centred approach by making the person and their story central to the event. Frank (2000), Kleinmann (1988) and others consider narrative as a means of being with others. This involves having an understanding of and ability to identify with the individual and the ability to be empathetic and caring toward that person. This mirrors a person-centred approach that promotes being in relation (having a good interpersonal relationship, valuing the self and others), being in social context (identifying and linking to things that are important in the context of the world the person lives in), being in place (identifying and working with organisational influences), and being with self (being aware of personal values in order to understand the values of others).

Narratives bridge the gap between what is known and how to apply that knowledge (Kalitzkus and Mathiessen, 2009). Narratives have the potential to promote self-reflection and aid professional development through enablement of reflexive practice. Combining person-centred care and narrative can potentially enable a more comprehensive approach to the development of an effective workplace culture where the communication qualities of narrative such as active listening, open questioning, and exploration are combined with the principles of engagement, enlightenment and emancipation to promote person-centredness and ensure the voice of the vulnerable older person is heard.

PROCESS AND OUTCOME EVALUATION

The chosen methodology of this study was action research (AR). This methodology was chosen because it can offer a way of generating knowledge that comes from practice. It is both collective and participatory and seeks to change practice. Winter (1998), talks about the researcher finding their 'authentic voice', but AR is also about all the participants of an AR project having a voice and that voice being heard. It is also about using that voice to question preconceived ideas and mores and to assert new ideas and ways of doing things. This voice needs to enable practitioners to be empowered where they are constantly challenging 'prescribed assumptions'. At the heart of AR is the development of a learning organisation where mutual learning occurs, in the case of residential care settings, between practitioners and residents. Winter (1998) believes that an educational process is implicit in AR and that there has to be an educational component built in or what Dewing (2010) calls 'active learning'. Active learning is concerned with ensuring that different 'ways of knowing' are privileged, that critical dialogue occurs and that combining these enables learning to occur for all in the workplace where people are encouraged to do things in a different way. The process of evaluation that occurred throughout the project, as part of the ongoing work-based learning activities, ensured that all the stakeholders involved had a voice in the process of change. The way that evaluation occurs in participatory AR is not predetermined, but reflects the approaches taken in implementing the practice change (McNiff, 2000). In this study evaluation was both ongoing to inform actions, happening at each work-based learning day, and as an overarching activity. The ongoing evaluation informed minor changes, or approaches, to overcome challenges that were seen during the implementation of the framework of narrative practice. The overarching evaluation was used to assess the effectiveness of the implementation, and also to look more globally at the challenges. Information gained from the evaluation was used at programme days with participants as a means of looking at the overall culture of care. The purpose of this overarching evaluation was to identify the way the implementation occurred and to consider the overall effectiveness of the implementation on the quality of life of the residents and the care practices of the staff.

STUDY PROGRESS AND KEY FINDINGS

The structure of the research study was based around three cycles. Essentially these were: (i) narrative practice and culture identification, (ii) developing narrative practice and (iii) working in a storied way. Identifying the culture and gaining an understanding of the framework of narrative practice was an ongoing exercise throughout the lifetime of the study. However, at the beginning of the study it was important to identify the present culture, and the basic assumptions about how care was carried out that both staff and residents held. This was essential so that staff could identify what an effective culture was. Staff employed a number of methods to do this, namely; creative expression, interviews with residents and observations of practice. Data gathered from this exploration were analysed and utilised to form the basis of developing action plans. Throughout the process staff utilised the framework of narrative practice to inform their discussions on identifying culture, developing strategies and working in a storied way. They took account of both the pillars of the framework and the operational elements in all their learning activities. Having identified what the present culture looked like in both units, staff next looked at developing strategies to use in the second action cycle, developing narrative ways of working. During the work-based reflective learning sessions, staff discussed the themes identified and critically examined them. They devised ways of using these themes, to inform improvements in the way care was carried out, and in the quality of the lived experience for the residents. Developing narrative ways of working on both units focused on interactions staff had and supports needed to maintain and implement good/effective narrative informed care. Staff worked with an action plan template (Figure 10.2) to outline the action plans and how they would attempt to achieve them. The 'working in a storied way' action cycle was concerned with implementing the strategies and ideas identified in the 'developing narrative ways of working' cycle in the practice setting. Staff used an action plan template to identify the

Action Plan Template
What do we want to achieve?
What parts of the framework does this link with?
What do we need to do to achieve that?
Do we need any additional resources? If so what are they and how can we get them?

Figure 10.2 Action planning themes.

approaches they needed to take, people they needed to engage with, and resources that were needed to address issues identified.

Overall while the staff on Unit 1 engaged well with the identification of the culture and development of the action plan, the implementation of these action plans proved problematic. Staff focused on a technical approach that placed value on using tools as a means of identifying resident experience. They did not utilise the information they collected in a critical way to change the care experience of the older adults or to challenge practice or culture. Rather they used it as simply another method of gathering and storing information that did ensure the care the residents received was safe and particular to them but that often occurred in a haphazard way depending on who was interacting with them.

By contrast, on Unit 2 staff engaged in a positive and proactive way with the identification of culture, development and implementation of action plans. All staff, residents and relatives were involved in the discussions that took place around the action plans and a participative and collaborative approach was used when implementing the plans. The staff critically reflected on the existing practice and used the information they had gathered to both inform change and develop strategies to help them deal with challenges identified and to improve the care experience for residents. In this way they achieved an emancipatory action approach both by increasing and developing their own knowledge and also by changing the practice setting and culture of care to ensure that the quality of life of the residents was improved.

The evaluation highlighted approaches that worked and barriers that hindered the implementation of the framework. It was a valuable tool for the participants as it formed part of the work-based learning reflective practice sessions and highlighted areas of practice and culture where change needed to take place.

This study was concerned with enabling healthcare staff to understand the life-world of older adults and to operationalise person-centred care through the use of narrative thus giving voice to this vulnerable group. During the implementation and overall evaluation of the study, key outcomes emerged in relation to the findings. The key outcomes from the implementation of this framework in practice are based on narrative knowing, being and doing and centred around the key outcomes of:

1. How people responded to change (narrative being).
2. The development of shared understandings (narrative knowing).
3. Intentional action (narrative doing).

How people responded to change, the development of shared understandings and intentional action are interrelated and interlinked.

Narrative being

Narrative being focused on engagement and communicative spaces. While engagement is seen as crucial to the AR process very little has been written about the difficulties of encouraging engagement within a participatory AR study (Snoeren and Frost, 2011). It was therefore necessary to look to the organisational culture literature to examine the way participants in this study responded to change (Herscovitch and Meyer, 2002; O'Donnell and Boyle, 2008; Machin, Fogarty and Bannon, 2009). Critically reflecting on the way participants responded to change during the study, it was evident, from the findings, that both units demonstrated enthusiasm and a desire to be engaged and involved in the study at the outset. This was supported by the clinical nurse managers in their roles as co-facilitators. In line with emotional support (Herscovitch and Meyer, 2002), they believed that change would be beneficial for both the residents and the staff. The findings show the way each unit engaged in the programme days mimicked the way they engaged with the residents on their units. Unit 2 embraced the philosophy of the Framework of Narrative Practice, used it to engage with the residents, and encouraged their participation in all decisions and planning of activities that occurred there. On Unit 1, staff were knowledgeable about the framework but did not fully utilise it in their interactions with the residents, but rather in a limited one to one basis which did not allow for any collaboration or shared decision-making. By enabling the opening of communicative spaces, opportunities were created for people to have their voices heard. This approach worked in different ways on the two units.

Narrative knowing

In this study the development of shared understanding was exhibited in the way staff took account of their knowledge of self and in their understanding of their knowledge of the identity of the residents. It was also manifest in the leadership styles in terms of power and organisational considerations. According to Frie (2011) our stories and narrative identity represents who we are and where we come from, in other words our values and beliefs. They are interwoven with those of others and our selfhood is situated and linked to the wider cultural context of community. It is therefore important to include the stories of all who live and work in a context in order to truly investigate that context. Understanding the interrelatedness of stories can enable the creation and development of communal under-standings (Frie, 2011).

Intentional action

Intentional action is an approach to attain a desired goal and is based on the belief that this is the best way to accomplish that goal (Burks, 2001). The Framework of Narrative Practice was conceptualised to provide guidance for staff to take intentional action when working with older people in residential care settings. In particular, its intent is to look at the narra-tive of the work or the culture, look at the narrative of the residents and the staff, and look at the narrative of the everyday care processes, with the aim of developing action that is intentional and creates meaning for the residents and the care staff. According to Popova (2014), intentionality is a process of interaction between agents, and it is through this inter-action that we ultimately define who we are. In the Framework of Narrative Practice the operational elements, narrative being, narrative knowing and narrative doing provided a structure for staff, to help them integrate the personal narrative of the resident with the narrative of their existing circumstances and environment. The study illustrates the impor-tance of ensuring that practice context is taken account of in the implementation of AR and also the importance of ensuring that narrative being, knowing and doing are clear and understandable for change to occur.

REFLECTIONS ON DOING PERSON-CENTRED RESEARCH AND BEING A PERSON-CENTRED RESEARCHER

The process of reflection is one that is said to help both researchers and practitioners define and explore issues that arise in their work (Taylor, 2003). It can be used to examine critically things that are going badly or to look at things that are going well and to see how that happened and what can be done to continue the trend. This is assisted by how we place ourselves in the world or according to Heidegger (1962) 'being-in-the-world'. Our being in the world therefore influences our understanding of the situation, and it is also shaped by how others involved perceive the event. Johns (2005) describes reflection as a way of reinforcing our sense of self and reflective practice, as defending the knowledge we possess of our self and our experiences. While Johns believes that a certain amount of anxiety is useful in reflective practice he considers too much fear as detrimental to both the person and the reflection. However, several theorists believe we have an urge as humans to become more than we are, to be more than the self we start with to become a more embodied self, one that will allow us to grow and flourish. I believe that rather than reinforcing our sense of self, for many, the process of reflection can cause the person to lose the self, that is, become someone they had not intended to be. So in order for me to enable others to reflect, it was necessary for me to firstly consider and reflect on both my own self and my identity as a researcher and a person. A challenge, for me, was the unsettling reality of reflective self identity and the need to be authentic within a cultural context. Several researchers have identified that change in self-identity can occur due to development or ageing or in response to some major life crisis or change in life role (Manzi, Vignoles and Regalia, 2010; Thomas, Levack and Taylor, 2014). It is true that novice researchers undertaking a PhD thesis are undertaking a process of change, both self-change and professional change. What is also true is that change is difficult and often disruptive. As a novice researcher, I had not anticipated this disruption, both to my self-identity and to my psyche. I had also not anticipated the challenges that would occur in the study due to this disruption within others.

This self-reflection enabled me to look critically at the engagement of staff in a new light, one where I could understand the reasons for some of the challenges that arose in the study, but also where I was able to stand back and realise that the way things were happening was because of the need for staff on some level to protect their own self-identity.

KEY LEARNING

The framework offers an interrelatedness between epistemological and ontological interpretations of narrative and a new method of developing knowledge. The theoretical foundations of the study and the methodology utilised enable a hermeneutic meaningfulness to be manifest, that provides a congruence between the aspirational intent of the framework and the tangible aspects of the practice culture. In practical terms, the framework outlines an approach that provides staff with a template to enable them to make sense of narrative experiences and to use that knowledge in the provision of person-centred care. This in turn will enable the voice of older adults to be heard and to be accounted for when assessing, planning, developing and implementing their care.

REFERENCES

Bochner, A. (2001) Narrative's virtues. *Qualitative Inquiry*, **7**, 131–157.

Buckley, C., McCormack, B. and Ryan, A. (2014) Valuing narrative in the care of older people: a framework of narrative practice for older adult residential care settings. *Journal of Clinical Nursing*, **23**, 2565–2577.

Burks, K.J. (2001) Intentional action. *Journal of Advanced Nursing*, **34**, 668–675.

Dewing, J. (2010) Moments of movement: active learning and practice development. *Nurse Education in Practice*, **10**, 22–26.

Frank, A.W. (2000) Illness and autobiographical work: dialogue as narrative destabilization. *Qualitative Sociology*, **23**, 135–156.

Frie, R. (2011) Identity, narrative, and lived experience after postmodernity: between multiplicity and continuity. *Journal of Phenomenological Psychology*, **42**, 46–60.

Frid, N., Ohlen, J. and Bergbom, I. (2000) On the use of narratives in nursing research. *Journal of Advanced Nursing*, **32**, 695–703.

Hardy, S., Gregory, S. and Ramjett, J. (2009) An exploration of intent for narrative methods of inquiry. *Nurse Researcher*, **16**, 7–19.

Heidegger, M. (1962) *Being and Time*. Blackwell Publishers, Oxford.

Herscovitch, L. and Meyer, J.P. (2002) Commitment to organizational change: extension of a three-component model. *Journal of Applied Psychology*, **87**, 474.

Johns, C. (2005) Expanding the gates of perception, in *Transforming Nursing Through Reflective Practice*, 2nd edition (eds C. Johns and D. Freshwater). Blackwell Science, Oxford. pp. 1–12.

Kalitzkus, V. and Matthiessen, P.F. (2009) Narrative-based medicine: potential, pitfalls, and practice. *The Permanente Journal*, **13**, 80.

Kleinman, A. (1988) *The Illness Narratives: Suffering, Healing, and the Human Condition*. Basic Books, New York.

Machin, M.A., Fogarty, G.J. and Bannon, S.F. (2009) Predicting employees' commitment to and support for organisational change. *The Australian Journal of Organisational Psychology*, **2**, 10–18.

Manzi, C., Vignoles, V.L. and Regalia, C. (2010) Accommodating a new identity: possible selves, identity change and well-being across two life-transitions. *European Journal of Social Psychology*, **40**, 970–984.

McCormack, B. and McCance, T. (2010) *Person-Centred Nursing: Theory, Models and Methods*. Wiley Blackwell, Oxford.

McNiff, J. (2000) *Action Research in Organisations*. Routledge, London.

O'Donnell, O. and Boyle, R (2008) *Understanding and Managing Organisational Culture: A Discussion Paper*. IPA, Dublin.

Popova, Y.B. (2014) Narrativity and enaction: the social nature of literary narrative understanding. *Frontiers in Psychology*, **5**, 895.

Snoeren, M. and Frost, D. (2011) Realising participation within an action research project on two care innovation units providing care for older people. *International Practice Development Journal* https://www.fons.org/Resources/Documents/Journal/Vol1No2/IPDJ_0102_03.pdf (accessed 1 February 2017).

Taylor, C. (2003) Narrating practice: reflective accounts and the textual construction of reality. *Journal of Advanced Nursing*, **42**, 244–51.

Thomas, E.J., Levack, W.M. and Taylor, W.J. (2014) Self-reflective meaning making in troubled times change in self-identity after traumatic brain injury. *Qualitative Health Research*, **23**, 1033–47.

Winter, R. (1998) Finding a voice–thinking with others: a conception of action research. *Educational Action Research*, **6**, 53–68.

Editors' Commentary

In this chapter Catherine Buckley presents an innovative and challenging research project that illustrates real engagement with a population that often don't have their voices adequately heard – older people living in residential care settings. It is somewhat ironic that the residential care/nursing home sector is one of the most heavily regulated care sectors in the western world; within this context, residents themselves continue to have the lesser 'say' in how the system works for them. Their views and comments form a minor part in the whole inspection and regulation processes and in the collection of evidence to demonstrate meeting (national) standards. While it is usual to engage with older people to inform the development of these standards, their views are often drowned out by the power of empirical evidence and macro policy, resulting in the person-centredness of these standards being questionable, i.e. whose personhood is being represented? The framework developed by Buckley, whilst complex, offers real insights into what some of the key dimensions of person-centredness need to look like in a residential care setting. Narrative as a methodology for framework development enables the constructs to be derived from multiple voices. As the author explains, voice in this case is not just the expression of words, but it represents an articulation of the core of personhood and what really matters to people. To do this in a systematic and meaningful way is challenging and Buckley's work demonstrates many of those challenges. The chapter also demonstrates the challenges of implementing changes in practice and doing so in a systematic way. We can all advocate for the importance of collaboration, inclusion and participation in person-centred research, but doing so in reality is challenging, messy, frustrating and sometimes successful! Buckley's work contrasts the power of the context over the success or otherwise of implementation/practice development activities and it also shows the need for different facilitation approaches to address these different contextual characteristics. It may be the case that in Unit 1, a more direct and intense facilitation relationship was needed by the facilitator - but would this have led to sustainable change? – it might have done but only in the short term. Learning from changes that have been less successful is important to advancing implementation science and this chapter/Buckley's work is important in that context also.

11 Promoting Health Across the Lifespan: A Systems Approach

Elisabeth Fosse, Steffen Torp and Ingun Stang

Reflective questions

1. How may national and municipal policies affect health among families with children?
2. Is there a difference between person-centred and people-centred healthcare?
3. In what ways may person-centred healthcare contribute in preventing social inequalities in health?

OVERVIEW OF THE STUDY

Norway, along with most European countries, has a long tradition as a welfare state. Even though the concept of the welfare state may vary across countries and be administered through various institutional arrangements, the basic idea regarding redistribution of resources among social groups remains at the core. Building health policy is a part of the building of welfare states.

The Ottawa Charter for Health Promotion was adopted in 1986 and shapes the foundation for health promotion theory and practice. The main focus of the charter is on the determinants of health, and the fundamental conditions and resources for health are described in the following way: peace, shelter, education, food, income, a stable ecosystem, sustainable resources, social justice and equity (World Health Organization, 1986).

The charter further emphasised the notion of empowerment, depicted as: 'a process of enabling people to increase control over, and to improve, their own health'. Tones and Green (2004) claimed that empowerment is the core concept of health promotion and that 'to be healthy is to be empowered'. The essence of empowerment is gaining mastery and control in life, at personal, organisational and community levels exemplified by Rappaport's (1984) classic empowerment definition: 'a process: the mechanism by which people, organisations, and communities gain mastery over their lives'. Empowerment is multifaceted, multileveled and influenced by context (Schulz *et al.*, 1995). Consequently, empowerment will take different forms for different people, organisations and settings (Rappaport, 1987). The empowerment perspective is essential to the whole of society, but is especially needed in settings where power imbalances do not favour underprivileged groups (Freire, 1972), and where people are being dependent on others for essential services and support (Stang, 1998). Although empowerment is divided into different analytical levels, the distinction between

---

Person-Centred Healthcare Research, First Edition. Edited by Brendan McCormack, Sandra van Dulmen, Hilde Eide, Kirsti Skovdahl and Tom Eide.

levels may to some degree be artificial, as different levels of empowerment may be inextricably intertwined (Tones and Green, 2004). Thus, health promotion practice and research call for compound actions clearly reflected and emphasised in political strategies.

In the Ottawa charter, five strategies to develop health promotion were outlined: build healthy public policy, create supportive environments, strengthen community actions, develop personal skills, and reorient health services.

Regarding the point of building healthy public policy, the World Health Organization (1986) states: 'Health promotion goes beyond healthcare. It puts health on the agenda of policy makers in all sectors and at all levels, directing them to be aware of the health consequences of their decisions and to accept their responsibilities for health. Health promotion policy combines diverse but complementary approaches including legislation, fiscal measures, taxation and organisational change. It is coordinated action that leads to health, income and social policies that foster greater equity'. This statement shows that in order to achieve the aims of the Ottawa charter, it is necessary to focus on the social determinants of health, which require intersectoral action.

Ottawa Charter-inspired health promotion has been squarely on the Norwegian political agenda for two decades. However, the national policy emphasis has shifted balance between strategies aimed at individuals and structural strategies. A new Public Health Act (PHA)[1] was introduced in Norway on January 1, 2012 (Ministry of Health and Care Services, 2011). The PHA establishes a new foundation for strengthening systematic public health work and structural strategies by the development of policies and planning for societal development based on regional and local challenges and needs.

The PHA underlines that health inequities arise from the societal conditions in which people are born, grow, live, work and age – the social determinants of health. Furthermore, it is stated that social inequities in health form a pattern of a gradient throughout society. Levelling up the gradient by action on the social determinants of health is a core public health objective and it is stated that fair distribution of societal resources is good public health policy. The principle of Health in All Policies (HiAP) implies that equitable health systems are important to public health, but health inequities arise from societal factors beyond healthcare. This implies that the impact on health must be considered when policies and action are developed and implemented in all sectors.

The SODEMIFA project[2] addresses the implementation of the Norwegian policy to level the social gradient in health. This will demand multisectoral action and a focus on the social determinants of health. Based on a life course perspective, the target group is families and children. Local governments have the main responsibility for services aimed at families and children.

The project has been studying local implementation processes, focusing on institutions at different levels. Within health promotion, national government mostly has so-called soft governing tools available to stimulate implementation of national policy targets. Local democracy provides local decision-makers the opportunity to prioritise between targets and local leaders of services will have to follow decisions made by local governments. Traditionally, municipalities are organised in sectors, which does not promote multisectoral collaboration.

The overall research question is: how do local governments handle the challenges of addressing the social determinants of health and the social gradient?

---

[1] The Norwegian term 'Folkehelse' has a wider connotation than the English term 'Public Health', as it includes both traditional Public Health and Health Promotion.

[2] The research project presented in this chapter is funded by the Norwegian Research Council project 'Addressing the social determinants of health: Multilevel governance of policies aimed at families with children' (Project no. 213841/H10).

This has been operationalised in the following questions:

1. How do local policy makers take part in formulating policies towards families and children?
2. Are the issues of levelling the social gradient addressed?
3. Do local policy makers support the principle of Health in All Policies?

The project has collected data by use of surveys and qualitative case studies in both regions and municipalities. Also public registry data has been used.

PRINCIPLES OF PERSON-CENTREDNESS GUIDING THE STUDY

This project focusing on policy and structural conditions (and not on individual persons per se) was not explicitly planned as a person-centred study. Nevertheless, the philosophical values of the study may be seen as consistent with philosophical principles of person-centredness as it for instance adopts a holistic view on health and is clearly not driven by a medical reductionist approach to public health (Williams and Grant, 1998; Leplege *et al.*, 2007).

Children and young people's well-being is strongly dependent upon the nature and quality of their families and family support systems, and the communities in which they live. These factors are in turn affected by the local, regional and national policy environment, which both shape and are shaped by cultural attitudes towards children and family life (Stegeman and Costongs, 2012). Michael Marmot refers to these as the conditions in which we are 'born, grow, live, work and age' (CSDH, 2008).

Children's early experiences and how they impact on their health have long-term consequences. Positive exposures in early life can bolster a child and young person's long-term health, and help them build a 'capital reserve' that can be of benefit throughout life, while negative exposures can undermine this. The factors that can lead to or undermine health are very similar to the factors that lead to social vulnerability. In all countries in the EU, children born into lower socio-economic classes have more physical and mental health problems and live shorter lives than children in higher socio-economic classes. The concept of the health gradient is closely related to this, and refers to the *systematic* correlation between the level of health and social status, and to the linear or step-wise decrease in health that comes with decreasing social position.

Our empirical point of departure was that social inequalities in health are also increasing in Norway. Inequality develops as a result of various socially patterned exposures and behaviours starting in early life and continue through later life stages. For example, associations established between low houshold income and inadequate housing (Braubach and Fairburn, 2010) and socio-economic conditions in the place of residence during childhood are associated with health in old age, independently of more recent conditions (Curtis and Riva, 2008). Access to green areas, natural environments and human and social services are related to positive mental well-being (O'Campo *et al.*, 2009). Early childhood development has far reaching societal effects with implications for health inequalities in adult life (Chen *et al.*, 2007). Biological and social determinants influence an individual's conception, pregnancy and birth. From birth a wide variety of environmental, economic and social determinants influence the individual's health. This continues through pre-school, school, education and training, employment, family creation, mid-life and retirement (World Health Organization, 2008).

In other words, a poor start to life increases the probability of adverse developmental outcomes and to worse health, behavioural and economic outcomes over the life course (Pillas and Suhrcke, 2009). To compound matters, differences in health at an early age are likely to lead to even greater differences in later life (Poulton *et al.*, 2002).

The Scandinavian welfare states are usually characterised as social democratic welfare states (Esping-Andersen, 1990). The 'social democratic regime' is characterised by its emphasis on solidarity and universal principles in the distribution of services. This includes a principle of redistribution of resources among social groups, mainly through a progressive tax system and entitlements for vulnerable groups. This is a system of emancipation, not only from the market, but also from the family. The result is a welfare regime with direct transfers to children and one which takes direct responsibility for the care of children, providing the conditions for women with families to engage in paid work. Women are encouraged to work and the welfare state is dependent on female participation in the labour market.

Lundberg *et al.* (2008a,b) show that although all rich nations have welfare programmes, there are clear cross-national differences with respect to their design and generosity. These differences are evident in national variations in poverty rates, especially among children and older people. The ways in which social policies are designed, as well as their generosity, are important for health. Hence, social policies are of major importance for how we can tackle the social determinants of health.

Lundberg (2009) states that welfare policies aiming to provide children and their families with a decent standard of living and schools of good quality among other things, should contribute to child health and well-being. Research shows a clear relationship between family policy generosity and the child poverty rate: countries with more generous family policies tend to have substantially lower child poverty rates. There is also a clear relationship between family policy generosity and infant mortality.

PROCESS AND OUTCOME EVALUATION

The project focuses on the implementation of the PHA. Even though the municipalities are obliged to implement the act, they have relatively extensive freedom in prioritising local policies and measures. The project has been studying both the process and the outcomes. Two surveys have been conducted among all Norway's municipalities, measuring the situation immediately before the act was adopted and the situation after 2 years. The survey data were linked to public registry data about the municipalities. The process has been studied by performing interview studies in a number of municipalities. The aim of these studies has been to understand how local processes may promote or prevent the implementation of the act.

STUDY PROGRESS AND/OR KEY FINDINGS/IMPACTS ON PERSONS, PEOPLE, POPULATIONS

In this chapter so far we have aimed to establish the link between policies and person-centredness. The implementation of the Norwegian PHA will have consequences for the health and well-being of children and their families.

When we look at the municipalities overall, the main conclusion is that they are in different places when it comes to implementing public health and health promotion policies. The responsibility for public health and health promotion is to a large degree still left to the health sector. Still, we observe a change towards increased awareness of the HiAP approach to reduce social inequalities.

For some municipalities, the PHA is overdue and they have been working to include health in plans and establish intersectoral working groups for many years. The majority of the municipalities have public health coordinators, whose role should be to coordinate public health work across sectors. However, many of them are located in the health sector in part-time positions. From this location, very remote from the level where decisions are made, the public health coordinator is not in the position to have an overview of local determinants of health, or the municipal needs for public health measures. Furthermore, placing these roles within the health services does not facilitate collaboration with other service-providing agencies in order to implement policies or include health in plans. To comply with the PHA and develop their overview of local determinants, municipalities must consider employing a public health coordinator as well as locating this role in the municipal administrative organisation. By localising the coordinator with the chief executive leaders' staff or in the staff of the planning agency, the opportunities actually to have a coordinating role increase, and would give the coordinator some authority in the municipal administrative organisation. To have a specialised function to coordinate will also be important in order to fulfil obligations to complete the health overviews and collaborate with the county and actors from civil society.

To increase the priority of health in all policies, there also needs to be explicit support – and even political pressure – from the national government. Our findings indicate that funding is important to incentivise municipalities to take on the new challenges in public health work. Funding is always a strong signal of priority, and so far the funding to the municipalities following the PHA has been scarce. In other words, the findings show a mixed picture. The studies indicate that few municipalities have come very far in implementing intersectoral policies to reduce social inequalities. On the other hand, the Norwegian welfare state is to a large extent based on universal policies and measures, rather than specific programmes. Many of the measures that have an impact on the health and well-being of children and families are already in place; such as day care of good quality, child healthcare, etc. Even though these are measures that could impact on health inequalities, there continues to be a lack of awareness about the importance of services such as these.

REFLECTIONS ON DOING PERSON-CENTRED RESEARCH AND BEING A PERSON-CENTRED RESEARCHER

According to Leplege *et al.* (2007), person-centredness is not very well defined and a variety of terms have been used interchangeably, such as patient-, client-, person- and individual-centred. Researchers and practitioners focusing specifically on public health and policy have used the term people- (Williams and Grant, 1998; South, White and Gamsu, 2013) and citizen-centred (Ambrose, Lenihan and Milloy, 2006). In their analysis of different meanings of the concept Leplege *et al.* (2007) describe four different conceptual pictures addressing person-centredness: the person's specific and holistic properties; the persons' difficulties in everyday life; participation and empowerment; and respect for the person 'behind' the impairment or disease. Both Leplege *et al.* (2007) and McCormack (2003) underline the importance of focusing on social policies and on adaptation of both physical and social environments. Norway's PHA focuses on how municipalities should structure their work to address social determinants, change social and physical environments and to secure participation and empowerment of its citizens.

Even though the SODEMIFA project has its main focus on the structural conditions for reducing social inequalities in health among families with children, we will argue that the project has a person-centred focus in line with what has been described above. HiAP is developed to raise awareness about the negative consequences of social inequalities in a life course approach. The aim of the policies is to develop measures to improve the quality of life for children and their families by addressing the social determinants.

McCormack (2003) points out that the organisation of practice, systems and approaches to work are key factors in person-centred practice and research, but that there has been little debate on how to address such issues in conducting research. The SODEMIFA project has an explicit focus on such issues. The use of both quantitative outcome measures and case studies with qualitative interviews and document analyses are also in line with principles of person-centred research (McCormack, 2003). The project's research group consists of researchers from many different disciplines such as political science, health promotion, epidemiology, nursing and pedagogy and thus securing a holistic and varied collection and interpretation of data.

REFERENCES

Ambrose, R., Lenihan, D.G. and Milloy, J. (2006) *Managing the Federation: A Citizen-Centred Approach.* Crossing the Bounderies National Council, Ottawa.

Braubach, M. and Fairburn, J. (2010) Social inequities in environmental risks associated with housing and residential location – a review of evidence. *European Journal of Public Health*, **20**, 36–42.

Chen, L., Yip, W., Chang, M-C. *et al.* (2007) The effects of Taiwan's National Health Insurance on access and health status of the elderly. *Health Economics*, **16**, 223–242.

CSDH (2008) *Closing the Gap in a Generation: Health Equity Through Action on the Social Determinants of Health.* Final Report of the Commission on Social Determinants of Health. World Health Organization, Geneva.

Curtis, S. and Riva, M. (2010) Health geographies II: complexity and health care systems and policy. *Progress in Human Geography*, **34**, 513–520.

Esping-Andersen, G. (1990) *The Three Worlds of Welfare Capitalism.* Polity Press, Cambridge.

Freire, P. (1972) *Pedagogy of the Oppressed.* Herder and Herder, New York.

Leplege, A., Gzil, F., Cammelli, M. *et al.* (2007) Person-centredness: conceptual and historical perspectives. *Disability and Rehabilitation*, **29**, 1555–1565.

Lundberg, O. (2009) How do welfare policies contribute to the reduction of health inequalities? *Eurohealth*, **15**, 24–27.

Lundberg, O., Yngwe, M.Å, Stjärne, M.K. *et al.*, for the NEWS Nordic Expert group. (2008a) The role of welfare state principles and generosity in social policy programs for public health: an international comparative study. *Lancet*, **372**, 1633–1640.

Lundberg, O., Yngve, M.Å., Stjärne, M.K. *et al.* (2008b) *The Nordic Experience: Welfare States and Public Health (NEWS).* Health equity studies No. 12. Centre for Health Equity Studies (CHESS). Karolinska Institutet, Stockholm University.

Ministry of Health and Care Services (2011) *Public Health Act, no. 29, 24-06-2011*, Oslo.

McCormack, B. (2003) Researching nursing practice: does person-centredness matter? *Nursing Philososophy*, **4**, 179–188.

O'Campo, P., Wheaton, B., Nisenbaum, R. *et al.* (2015) The Neighbourhood Effects on Health and Well-being (NEHW) study. *Health and Place*, **31**, 65–74.

Pillas, D. and Suhrcke, M. (2009) *Assessing the Potential or Actual Impact on Health and Health Inequalities of Policies Aiming to Improve Early Child Development (ECD) in England.* Background Report to Marmot Review.

Poulton, R., Caspi, A., Milne, B.J. *et al.* (2002) Association between children's experience of socioeconomic disadvantage and adult health: a life-course study. *Lancet*, **360**, 1640–1645.

Rappaport, J. (1984) Studies in empowerment: introduction to the issue. *Community Mental Health Review*, **3**, 1–7.

Rappaport, J. (1987) Terms of empowerment/exemplars of prevention: toward a theory for community psychology. *American Journal of Community Psychology*, **15**, 121–148.

Stegeman, I and Costongs, C. (eds) (2012) *Levelling the Gradient in Child and Adolescent Health in Europe: Evidence, Policy and Practice*. Eurohealthnet, Brussels.

Schulz, A.J., Israel, B.A., Zimmerman, M.A. and Checkoway, B.N. (1995) Empowerment as a multi-level construct: perceived control at the individual, organizational and community levels. *Health Education Research*, **10**, 309–327.

South, J., White, J. and Gamsu, M. (2013) *People-Centred Public Health*. Policy Press, Bristol.

Stang, I. (1998) *Makt og bemyndigelse – om å ta pasient og brukermedvirkning på alvor [Power and empowerment - on taking patient and person participation seriously]*. Universitetsforlaget, Oslo.

Tones, K. and Green, J. (2004) *Health Promotion. Planning and Strategies*. Sage, London.

Williams, B. and Grant, G. (1998) Defining 'people-centredness': making the implicit explicit. *Health and Social Care in the Community*, **6**, 84–94.

World Health Organization (1986) The Ottowa Charter for Health Promotion: First International Conference on Health Promotion, Ottawa, 21 November 1986. http://www.who.int/healthpromotion/conferences/previous/ottawa/en/(accessed 1 February 2017).

Editors' Commentary

We are delighted to include a chapter in this book that focuses on health promotion and in particular, a chapter that concentrates on the systems level. As the authors have highlighted, whilst most health systems have a mandate for and a focus on promoting health, in reality 'managing' illness tends to dominate. In countries such as Norway, where healthcare is provided free to the population (paid for through taxation) and where a high proportion of the GDP is invested in healthcare, then one would expect health outcomes to be positive. But as Fosse and colleagues point out, Norway, like many other countries has a changing demographic and even in such a well-resourced welfare system promoting positive health is challenging. Fosse and colleagues provide a convincing argument for their work being viewed through a person-centred lens. The World Health Organization (WHO) in their *Global Strategy on Integrated People-centred Health Services 2016–2026* (http://apps.who.int/iris/bitstream/10665/180984/1/WHO_HIS_SDS_2015.20_eng.pdf?ua=1&ua=1) explicitly locate their strategic framework in person-centred values. They define people-centred care as:

> *an approach to care that consciously adopts individuals', carers', families' and communities' perspectives as participants in, and beneficiaries of, trusted health systems that respond to their needs and preferences in humane and holistic ways. People-centred care also requires that people have the education and support they need to make decisions and participate in their own care. It is organized around the health needs and expectations of people rather than diseases (p. 4).*

They also define person-centred care as:

> *care approaches and practices that see the person as a whole with many levels of needs and goals, with these needs coming from their own personal social determinants of health (p. 4).*

The research being undertaken by Fosse and colleagues is clearly in line with this strategy and challenges existing health and welfare systems to not take health for granted but to consider the expectations of individuals, communities and populations also. The authors argue the case for persons to be viewed holistically and thus there is a need for all healthcare practitioners to think about health promoting aspects of their work – something that remains a challenge to many healthcare practitioners. Therefore, whilst Fosse and colleagues are (understandably) critical of health promotion coordinators being placed within the health sector, there may be benefits to this in the way these coordinators can challenge existing attitudes to health promotion and its (lack of) priority in healthcare delivery systems. If persons are to be viewed holistically by healthcare practitioners, then the health promotion role of all healthcare professionals needs to be recognised and developed more actively. Research such as this reported here has the potential to influence such developments.

12 How Knowledge Developed Through Ethnography May Inform Person-Centred Healthcare Practices

Kristin Briseid, Astrid Skatvedt and Brendan McCormack

Reflective questions

1. What kind of knowledge may foster the development of care contexts conducive to person-centred practices?
2. What kind of knowledge may contribute to individualised care, including attention to needs for coping as well as needs for care and protection?
3. How can ethnographic research contribute to such knowledge?

INTRODUCTION

In this chapter, we discuss how ethnographic research approaches may be suitable for knowledge development in person-centred healthcare practices (PCP). We illustrate our argument with empirical examples from an ethnographically oriented research project we were involved in between 2012 and 2015. The project concerned Norwegian municipal healthcare services for older people living with mental health issues.

BACKGROUND

Ethnography denotes a research methodology based on observation of events and actions in natural environments (Hammersley and Atkinson, 1983/1996). It often implies that the researcher stays with people in different ways and adopts several roles: as a participant observer, as an observing participant, as an interviewer or someone with whom to make small-talk (Hammersley and Atkinson, 1983/1996). An ideal in analytic work is to achieve as rich or 'thick' field descriptions as possible (Geertz, 1973).

We draw attention here to two distinct methodological advantages of ethnography that we consider important in a PCP setting. We ask whether each advantage may match well with a given type of knowledge required in light of corresponding aspects of PCP as a healthcare ideal. The first concerns ethnography's potential for context awareness, where the researcher is also a part of the context (Hammersley and Atkinson, 1983/1996; Whyte, 1993). This may

---

Person-Centred Healthcare Research, First Edition. Edited by Brendan McCormack, Sandra van Dulmen, Hilde Eide, Kirsti Skovdahl and Tom Eide.

foster knowledge about how context influences healthcare, which matches with a PCP-related demand for awareness about contexts of care.

The second concerns the potential for bringing researchers close to the everyday lives of persons to understand what happens there (Schatzman and Strauss, 1973; Hammersley and Atkinson, 1983/1996). Closeness may enable knowledge development concerning needs and interests that might otherwise remain undisclosed. One example is the possibility of gaining relevant data from experienced key informants that would otherwise remain hidden (Hammersley and Atkinson, 1983/1996). This advantage matches with a PCP-related demand for individualised care approaches. We claim that individualised care requires acknowledgement that human needs and interests are composite and include both needs for 'coping' and needs for 'care and protection'.

THE TERM PCP – AND A TENSION CONCERNING A VIEW OF HUMANITY?

Healthcare practitioners seeking to facilitate PCP consider the balancing of different values: partly competing care values and partly organisational values (Woods, 2001).

We therefore consider it important to study how different aspects of PCP relate to each other as they may reflect care values that come into conflict when realised in practice. We also consider it important to study how different aspects of PCP relate to interests rooted in influential organisational or societal forces. Such forces may push healthcare practices towards certain solutions to conflict between PCP values. PCP concerns treating persons as 'ends in themselves' rather than as means to another's end (McCormack, 2004). PCP may therefore depend on capacity to protect healthcare from becoming colonialised by forces that favour understanding of 'good care' consonant with only some carefully selected PCP values.

Rosemari Eliasson-Lappalainen (1995) claims that good care depends on the capacity to keep alive an unresolvable tension. It concerns views of humanity and the relationship between two principles. One principle denotes respect for the individual's will and capacity for coping. The other denotes respect for dependence of persons on others. Mia Vabø argues that in times of economic austerity, there is a danger of suppression of the tension, and that care practices founded in confined views of humanity may evolve (Vabø, 2007).

We draw attention to a potential tension between PCP values, and between PCP values and organisational values. Inspired by Eliasson and Vabø, we see it as concerning the relationship between two care principles. Here, we call them (1) the 'coping principle' and (2) the 'dependency principle'. The first embodies valuing respect for persons' strengths and resources, nourishing capacity for agency and involvement in decision-making, and respecting persons as autonomous beings whose empowerment is crucial. Among the PCP attributes mentioned in the literature, respectfulness, empowerment and sharing decision-making reflect this principle (Morgan and Yoder, 2012; Sjögren *et al.*, 2012).

By the 'dependency principle', we mean respecting persons as vulnerable, dependent on others and on society. It implies recognising their need for care and protection when they cannot or will not take care of themselves, and/or when their inclination towards involvement is weak. As we see it, the focus in the PCP literature on relationships and social environments, and on individualisation of care, reflects this principle. Individualisation requires understanding of the person's situation, and of his or her ability or desire to make decisions and take control of his or her care (Morgan and Yoder, 2012).

In the following sections, we will briefly describe a Norwegian action research project we were involved in, and present empirical examples from that project. We do so in an attempt to shed light on our overarching argument concerning ethnography's capacity for informing PCP.

OUR RESEARCH CONCERNING OLDER PEOPLE'S MENTAL HEALTH

The action research project took place between 2012 and 2015 and concerned municipal mental health services for people over the age of 65. It was located at the University College of Southeast Norway, and received funding from the Research Council of Norway. Part of its background was a conclusion from an evaluation report from the Research Council, concerning the National Action Plan for Mental Health. Norwegian healthcare services had often overlooked older people with mental health problems (Norges Forskningsråd, 2009).

The original project design was not ethnographic. It prescribed data collection through individual and group interviews: with patients, care partners, healthcare professionals and leaders. We followed a pre-elaborated interview guide focusing on experiences with collaboration between health services and service users and care partners. Healthcare professionals helped us to recruit interview participants.

An important reason why the project relied heavily on ethnography was a realisation that its embedding in the municipal organisation was weak. A municipal leader, who had originally cooperated with the University College on the project proposal, had quit. The new leader was unfamiliar with the project. Time pressure complicated the possibilities for the home-based services to inform patients and solicit consent for interviews. We gradually saw the project as 'forgotten' in the municipality. Therefore, in December 2012, to become more visible to stakeholders and potential participants, we decided to embark on ethnographic fieldwork using participant observation. We began in the home-based services and the mental health team (MHT), having received ethical approval from the Norwegian Social Science Data Services.

Rapid recruitment advances followed this 'ethnographic turn'. It also coloured our mindset about the individual interviews, so that the pre-elaborated interview guide became less important. To ethnographers, it is an ideal to permit the participants' 'own story' to be told, and to let theory 'take the back seat' – at least in the initial phases of a study (Holstein and Gubrium, 1997). We opted for more open, informal conversations and tried to enable situations where each individual could present his or her account of the issues experienced as important in their contact (or lack of it) with the municipality.

The 'ethnographic turn' implied travelling around in a car with the home care nurses and seeing them with persons in their own homes. We attended meetings and listened to discussions in the home-based services and in the MHT. Later, we worked ethnographically at the service office (where decisions about services are made), among administrative leaders, in the political committee for health and care and the community council. We carried out field talks and structured, interview-like conversations. Following Lofland and Lofland, the latter often took the form of 'intensive interviewing': guided talks aimed at achieving a rich, detailed material (1984, p. 12). We wrote field notes during or after observation sessions.

Below, we present data we achieved by working this way, and try to show how context awareness and getting close may have facilitated our possibilities for developing knowledge suited for informing PCP.

ETHNOGRAPHIC DATA ABOUT CARE CONTEXT – AND ABOUT OTHERWISE POSSIBLY HIDDEN NEEDS AND INTERESTS

In a MHT meeting, the team members discussed an experience that too many patients needed help relative to the number of team professionals. The following material is an edited excerpt from the field notes.

The leader, Liv[1], concluded by stating:

OK, I will think about what we can do. Because in years to come, our capacity challenges will probably just increase. More patients than we will have employees to attend to will continue being referred here.

Sigrid raised her hand:

I think it could be worth a try to plan the ending of our relationship with service users. My experience is that positive recourses [in the service users] can be triggered if people know from the outset about a date when their relationship with the professional will end. A lot of research supports this.

Renate followed up:

Yes, I agree. You mobilise your own forces that way. You experience that the professional reinforces your ability to cope. It is as if the professional tells the service user, 'I am not your lifeline. You are your own lifeline'.

Karen asked if she could speak. Her voice quivered slightly as she said that mental health illness was unpredictable, and that the suggested routine would therefore not always work.

We must remember we are safeguarding legislation. Our responsibility is not just to treat people (…). I think the regional governor will disapprove if we initiate such a practice here.

The excerpt displays healthcare professionals seeking to balance values. It illustrates a concern for PCP values as empowerment and individualisation. It also reflects the impact of organisational or societal values. Apparently, Sigrid's view reflects concern for the 'coping principle', while Karen seems to be defending the 'dependency principle'. Based on our impression of Karen's body language, our interpretation was that defending the 'dependency principle' was emotionally hard.

Later, we asked Sigrid about her positive view on 'setting a date'. She said:

You depend totally on having good people around you when you are in a difficult mental health situation. But are we just to forget about the role of family and things like that?

We also asked Karen about her scepticism. She said:

Some of our patients do not have anyone else around them. Their social network is often very meagre, or they don't have one at all. They may have only us. Just knowing we are here, that they

---

[1] All the names of research participants used in this chapter are pseudonyms.

have an appointment with us... It may help them stay stable – in a situation where they otherwise would become hospitalised. (...) It won't work for everyone to plan for an end. It may work for some, but not everyone.

We asked two MHT leaders about their opinions. Both said they favoured a 'planning for the end' line, as a method for prioritising resources. Liv said:

If we plan for ending relationships with more service users, it means that more service users may receive help.

The other leader, Tone, emphasised that anyone who phoned the team would be able to talk with someone even after the relationship had formally ended.

Some weeks later, the suggestion came up again in a meeting. No one argued against it then, except for one team member, Elisabeth, who commented, without receiving any response: '(...) But...there has not been agreement on this issue in the team earlier, has there?'

Elisabeth's comment seems to convey a perception of a shift in balance occurring over time in the team. It seemed to pass unnoticed. As ethnographers, we achieved concrete descriptions of its whereabouts. The ethnographic potential for context awareness facilitated data about the relationship between the shift and economic austerity, and with an expectation of future economic deterioration. Ethnographic closeness facilitated knowledge about perspectives (associated with the 'dependency principle') that might otherwise possibly have remained undisclosed to us. Our interpretation was that a tension between PCP values became imbalanced and lost some of its original force. The 'coping principle' increased in prominence at the cost of the 'dependency principle'. Apparently, a background of organisational values, related to economic austerity, fitted better with a strong 'coping principle'.

DISCUSSION

With reference to the data excerpt above, subsequent sections will discuss how ethnography may foster context awareness and closeness, and how this again may be valuable when knowledge development aims at informing PCP practices.

Context awareness

A key point in the PCP literature is that PCP depends not only on the characteristics of healthcare providers. It needs support from the context of care, including an organisational level (McCormack and McCance, 2010; Morgan and Yoder, 2012). Consequently, healthcare stakeholders seeking to influence care contexts in such ways as to promote PCP, may need knowledge about societal forces that mark the context of care. The MHT meeting story illustrated this well. Apparently, Karen's defence for the 'dependency principle' lost legitimacy due to an experience of mismatch between available personnel and number of service users. It also lost legitimacy due to an apparently taken for granted expectation of increased demand for services, and presumably also because leaders did not support this position.

The way the team members referred to external, apparently authoritative, sources in defence of each principle is also interesting. Karen referred to legislation and the regional governor and Sigrid referred to research. Such data may serve as hints about how the capacity to 'keep tension alive' may depend on how the regional governor safeguards legislation.

The capacity to keep tension alive may also depend on the knowledge type researchers develop and convey to professionals.

Other methods, such as qualitative interviews or statistical surveys, could also have provided data about contextual conditions. An advantage of ethnography, however, is that it helps the researcher focus accurately on the contextual aspects that seem most salient to participants' everyday practices. The researcher may interact with participants over time and in different settings. This facilitates a collaborative practice with participants regarding data development and analytical work. Further, the concrete descriptions of how context influences practice may make ethnographically developed knowledge particularly suitable as 'maps' (Smith, 2005), or practical guides to 'finding the way' in a system or society – in order to promote PCP.

Getting close – discovering hidden needs and interests

The PCP literature often describes the term PCP and its related terms as having emerged due to experiences with healthcare practices that fail to have the interests of *persons* at their centre (Mead and Bower, 2000; McCormack, 2004; Morgan and Yoder, 2012). As we see it, the raison d'être of PCP is therefore that healthcare stakeholders and researchers may need a term like PCP when seeking to distinguish persons' needs from other needs/interests. Without such help, visions may more easily become blurred.

Societal forces that are pressuring healthcare systems towards suppressing tension may foster such blurring in at least two ways. One is by nourishing reluctance among people to express with certainty their real felt needs or interests. For example, vocabularies suited for descriptions of needs and interests considered unwanted in an economic perspective may be discarded as non-authoritative. A consequence may be that people cease voicing such needs. In a PCP context, this constitutes a challenge. It may for example hamper the capacity on the part of researchers and healthcare stakeholders to grasp the compositeness of the experienced needs of persons. A risk is that healthcare stakeholders and researchers end up basing work on needs perceptions rooted in the forces that are pushing towards confinement.

The MHT story illustrates how such forces, associated with economic austerity, contributed to reluctance about voicing certain perspectives. Gradually, it became more challenging to voice persons' dependency-related needs. Being close to this development made us as researchers attentive to the potential salience, in a PCP perspective, of such weakly voiced or silenced perspectives. Our impression was that silence or weak voicing did not necessarily indicate that a perspective was irrelevant to the team members or to their service users, nor that it was irrelevant in a PCP perspective. It might just as well be a result of the impact of economic austerity.

There is also a second way whereby forces pushing towards confinement may cause blurred visions and reduced capacity to distinguish persons' needs from other needs: these forces may influence the researchers' and healthcare stakeholders' frame of understanding. When developing research questions and conceptual categories for a statistical survey from a distance, there is for example, a possibility that questionnaires end up reflecting dominant societal understandings of persons' needs. This may lead to knowledge development founded in confined views of humanity – which in turn may colour the needs perceptions upon which healthcare stakeholders base their practices.

Ethnographers are not immune to this. Societal forces influence their frame of understanding, too. However, ethnographers dispose of methodological resources that may mitigate their impact on knowledge development. One is the access to data not only about what people say, but also about what they do, the context of where they do it, and about what they seem to feel about interaction and actions (Hammersley and Atkinson, 1983/1996). A second is the ideal of permitting participants' stories to take precedence over academic theories and concepts when defining research questions (Holstein and Gubrium, 1997, p. 177). Finally, ethnographers are encouraged to treat their personal reactions to events as potential entry points to a broadened understanding of how the field of study relates to society wherein it is embedded (Narayan, 1993, p. 197).

Such resources provide knowledge development processes with a certain potential for increased robustness. This may be valuable given a PCP-related aim of distinguishing persons' needs from other needs, and of enabling healthcare stakeholders to prioritise the former.

CONCLUSION

Pragmatic reasons brought about the ethnographic turn of our research about PCP to older people with mental health issues. Nevertheless, the additional advantages ethnography brought with it, may serve to illuminate a general argument about how knowledge developed ethnographically may inform PCP practices. We have claimed that PCP requires capacity to keep alive a tension between potentially contradictory principles for good care. The tension is important because care practices embodying confined views of humanity may otherwise evolve. These may fail to address the compositeness of persons' actual needs.

KEY LEARNING

The ethnographic potential for context awareness fosters an understanding of concrete steps that may be taken to develop care contexts conducive to PCP. We were particularly concerned with how care contexts could become conducive or hostile to keeping tension alive. Closeness through ethnographic work contributed to fostering understanding of aspects of persons' needs and interests that may otherwise have remained hidden to the gaze of researchers. Overall, therefore, our key learning is that the potential for closeness and contextual awareness will often make ethnography a good fit for knowledge development aimed at informing PCP.

REFERENCES

Eliasson-Lappalainen, R. (1995) *Forskningsetik och perspektivval [Research ethics and the choice of perspectives]*. Studentlitteratur, Lund.

Geertz, C. (1973) *The Interpretation of Cultures*. Basic Books, New York.

Hammersley, M. and Atkinson, P. (1983/1996) *Ethnography: Principles in Practice*. Routledge, London.

Holstein, J.A. and Gubrium, J.F. (1997) *The New Language of Qualitative Method*. Oxford University Press, New York.

Lofland, J. and Lofland, L.H. (1984) *Analyzing Social Settings: A Guide to Qualitative Observation and Analysis*. Wadsworth, Belmont.

McCormack, B. (2004) Person-centredness in gerontological nursing: an overview of the literature. *Journal of Clinical Nursing*, **13**(s1), 31–38.

McCormack, B. and McCance, T. (2010) *Person-Centred Nursing: Theory and Practice*. Wiley Blackwell, Oxford.

Mead, N. and Bower, P. (2000) Patient-centredness: a conceptual framework and review of the empirical literature. *Social Science and Medicine*, **51**, 1087–1110.

Morgan, S. and Yoder, L.H. (2012) A concept analysis of person-centered care. *Journal of Holistic Nursing*, **30**, 6–15.

Narayan, K. (1993) How native is a 'native' anthropologist? *American Anthropologist*, **95**, 671–676.

Norges Forskningsråd (2009) Evaluering av Opptrappingsplanen for psykisk helse (2001-2009).

Schatzman, L. and Strauss, A. (1973) *Field Research: Strategies for a Natural Sociology*. Prentice-Hall, Englewood Cliffs.

Sjögren, K., *et al.* (2012) Psychometric evaluation of the Swedish version of the Person-Centered Care Assessment Tool (P-CAT). *International Psychogeriatrics*, **24**, 406.

Smith, D.E. (2005) *Institutional Ethnography: A Sociology for People*. AltaMira, Lanham.

Vabø, M. (2007) Organisering for velferd: hjemmetjenesten i en styringsideologisk brytningstid. Oslo, Norsk institutt for forskning om oppvekst, velferd og aldring. Avhandling (dr.philos.) - Universitetet i Oslo, 2007.

Whyte, W.F. (1993) *Street Corner Society. The Social Structure of an Italian Slum*. University of Chicago Press, Chicago.

Woods, R.T. (2001) Discovering the person with Alzheimer's disease: cognitive, emotional and behavioural aspects. *Aging and Mental Health*, **5**, 7–16.

Editors' Commentary

In earlier chapters of this book, issues of ontological and epistemological positioning (Chapter 3) and the 'being' of a person-centred researcher (Chapter 4) were addressed. Issues about methodological eclecticism, values clarification, engagement and connectedness were identified as being important in person-centred research. The methodological discussion presented in this chapter brings many of these issues into stark reality. Briseid and colleagues use their experiences of engaging in a research project with older people experiencing mental health issues as a focus to consider many of the methodological challenges experienced when engaging in person-centred research. The project in question had the intention of being a participatory action research project informed by emancipatory principles, but from the outset this became problematic. Again, it is not unusual for the intentions in the pre-determined design for action research not to come to fruition in the implementation of the said design – the challenges of action research are well rehearsed in the literature. Did Briseid and colleagues make the right decisions when faced with the dilemmas they outline? Was the 'ethnographic turn' the right thing to do or should they have re-grouped the stakeholders in the municipality and re-established the action research intent? In many ways this is a rhetorical question and dependent on a variety of factors, not least of which, the 'being' of the researchers. However, in the context of this book, the question is far from rhetorical as the decisions made reflect what McCormack and McCance (2017) have referred to as 'engaging authentically' – an ethical stance of being real in a situation, reflecting the context of the situation and respecting the 'being of the other'. An easy solution would have been to convince the new leadership that the project as conceived had to proceed as plan, but the risk to relationships and respect for research as an empowering activity would be great. Instead, the ethnographic turn created an opportunity to develop more meaningful relationships with all the stakeholder groupings involved and to develop a deep understanding of the differing underpinning values and agendas that influenced their decisions and actions. Doing this has raised new insights into understanding why person-centredness might be a challenge to implement in some situations as well as the relationship between macro and micro level agendas in a healthcare context. The 'action' that resulted may not have been that of bringing about systems or care process changes, but that is not what action necessarily means in the context of action research. Achieving 'enlightenment' is an essential process in emancipatory action research and is action in itself. As the authors demonstrate, the enlightenment achieved in terms of understanding the potential contradictory forces that prevent person-centredness from being realised is action in itself. The chapter does however challenge the wisdom of predetermining the detail of action research cycles of action in order to satisfy the criteria for securing research funding. There is a big challenge here to research funders and how they understand action research in the context of being person-centred. This is an area that needs further consideration and engagement by the research community as a whole.

McCormack, B. and McCance, T. (eds) (2017) *Person-centred Practice in Nursing and Healthcare: Theory and Practice*. Wiley Blackwell, Oxford.

13 Person-Centred Technology-Supported Interventions

Sandra van Dulmen, Espen Brembo, Janne Dugstad
and Hilde Eide

Reflective questions

1. How can technology uplift today's healthcare services?
2. Are technology-supported innovations person-centred?
3. How can technology enhance personhood?

INTRODUCING TECHNOLOGY-BASED HEALTHCARE SERVICES

Krijgsman and Klein Wolterink (2012) make a distinction between technology-supported healthcare interventions (eHealth) along three dimensions: the care process (in which the technology becomes embedded), the user, and the technology. Along the line of the care process, technology can be used to support or improve health and healthcare. In terms of the user, the authors refer to the end user for whom the technology-supported intervention is developed, i.e. the service user, the health professional or others. In terms of technology, different interventions can be identified, varying from web-applications to home automation/smart home solutions. What the latter interventions have in common is that they all use new information and communication technology (ICT), in particular internet technology, to support and enhance health and healthcare. An additional and relevant categorisation of ICT-supported interventions can be made by incorporating their specific function or aim; an intervention can be developed to support the care process (e.g. electronic medical records or an app for making an appointment with a doctor), to reach the public (e.g. through internet-based education, prevention and campaigns) or to complement or replace traditional healthcare interventions (e.g. psychotherapy online or telemonitoring). By combining these functions with the characteristics of the pursued end-users, Krijgsman and Klein Wolterink were able to categorise all possible interventions.

In view of the current paradigm shift towards person-centred healthcare in general and person-centred technology-supported care in particular, there is, however, a need to also weigh new technology-supported interventions in terms of the level of person-centredness. In other words, an answer should be sought to the question as to what extent different technology-supported interventions support and integrate the individual's healthcare needs,

---

Person-Centred Healthcare Research, First Edition. Edited by Brendan McCormack, Sandra van Dulmen,
Hilde Eide, Kirsti Skovdahl and Tom Eide.
© 2017 John Wiley & Sons Ltd. Published 2017 by John Wiley & Sons Ltd.

preferences and values. This chapter therefore aims to provide input for this additional dimension by presenting and evaluating three technology-supported interventions in different stages of development (finished, ongoing and being set up) along the lines of person-centredness. This input is meant to turn the functional descriptive categorisation by Krijgsman and Klein Wolterink (2012) into a living model that may serve to capture and monitor the fast expanding world of technology-supported interventions. Such an expanded model may provide a clear overview of the types of technology-supported interventions that have already evolved into a set of real person-centred technology-supported interventions and for which category more effort is needed to get there.

TECHNOLOGY-SUPPORTED INTERVENTIONS: EXAMPLES FROM THREE STUDIES

The interventions presented here are just three of many examples of technology-supported interventions that are being developed as part of the technologisation of today's healthcare. The examples include: an evidence-based therapy for people with long-term conditions provided in an innovative way, a safety service for vulnerable people and their caregivers, and a support tool for empowering service users who face difficult healthcare decisions.

Web-based, self-management enhancing interventions for patients with long-term conditions

Three web-based interventions were developed and tested for people living with long-term conditions based on cognitive behavioural therapy (CBT) and acceptance and commitment therapy (ACT) principles. These interventions aimed at increasing persons' self-management skills and quality of life (Oerlemans *et al.*, 2011; Kristjánsdóttir *et al.*, 2011, 2013a, 2013b; Nes *et al.*, 2012, 2013, 2014). When developing the interventions, the Medical Research Council framework for complex interventions was used involving four separate stages (Craig *et al.*, 2008): development, feasibility and piloting, evaluation, and implementation. The feasibility and efficacy of these interventions were investigated for people with irritable bowel syndrome (in a randomised controlled trial), chronic widespread pain (randomised controlled trial) and type 2 diabetes (feasibility study) with 76, 140 and 15 persons, respectively. In each study the intervention group participants completed e-diaries during several weeks on a PDA (personal digital assistant) or smartphone and received personalised, situational feedback based on their input on the same day. In the e-diaries, the participants registered activities, emotions and pain cognitions three times daily using the mobile device by choosing between predefined options and scales. A therapist had immediate access to this information through a secured website and used the situational information to formulate and send a personalised message to the participant with the aim of stimulating effective self-management in coping with the current situation. The web-based interventions appeared feasible, acceptable and supportive. In the short and medium term, the interventions also appeared to promote self-management.

Digital night surveillance of persons with dementia

Digital surveillance technology was developed and implemented in services providing care to people living with dementia (Nilsen *et al.*, 2016). The technology included sensors on doors and in electronic security blankets (on mattresses) used during the night, and a web-based portal to facilitate communication via traditional personal computers (PCs) as well as mobile devices like tablets and smartphones. Most of the local health services already had some welfare technology installed, such as alarm systems, and the novelty of the new systems was tied to the web-based portal into which different technological applications can be connected and administered. In this way, technology in different categories and from different producers can function together and be programmed to individual persons' needs. Initially, decisions were made regarding what type(s) of technology was suitable for the individual user, and alarm settings were customised for each person. Alterations can be made based on for instance variations in needs during the day or due to the progression of a disease. An alarm will go off when an incident happens and the technology is programmed for the individual person. The system is programmed to send alarm messages to dedicated personnel, and they receive an alarm on the device that has been chosen by their municipality or service: a smartphone, iPad or PC, or a combination. They switch off the alarm as they check on the user. Most home care service residents are in need of night supervision. They are living with dementia and tend to get up at night and wander, which has been described as one of the behaviours that is difficult to manage (Lai and Arthur, 2003). Night surveillance in one form or another (face-to-face or technology based) is necessary to detect 'night wanderers' and guide them back to bed in order to prevent confusion and anxiety, avoid falling and injuries, and protect other residents from being disturbed and becoming frightened during the night. In the Digital Night Surveillance project, the sensors in blankets and on doors detect and send a signal when a person gets out of bed during the night and when the person leaves the room. The persons with dementia are only passively using the technology, whereas the nursing staff responsible for administrating patient data, checking equipment and receiving alarms are actively using it. The implementation requires strategies for education and training, as well as for establishment of new routines, quality assurance procedures, initial adoption and upscaling.

MY HIP: A WEB-BASED INFORMATION AND SUPPORT TOOL FOR PERSONS WITH HIP OSTEOARTHRITIS

People confronted with hip osteoarthritis need to adapt to the consequences of their illness and to get acquainted with different ways to manage these, related to medical aspects, emotion handling and changes in life roles. Medical management includes monitoring symptoms, changing health behaviours, and working with health professionals. Emotional management concerns dealing with the emotional consequences of having a long-term condition, such as anger, guilt, despair and frustration. Role management is about coming to terms with a change in life role, i.e. from 'healthy' to 'sick', and from 'providing' to 'being cared for'. Accomplishing these challenges requires a considerable degree of informational, behavioural, emotional, and social support for the individual person (Murray, 2009). Well-designed internet interventions have promising effects on users, including enhancing knowledge, self-efficacy, perceived social support, health behaviours and clinical outcomes (Murray, 2008). Osteoarthritis of the hip is a prevalent source of pain and disability in older people and there is currently no therapy available to stop or reverse the progression of osteoarthritis. Treatment includes conservative approaches and surgical joint replacement in suitable individuals (Zhang *et al.*, 2008). Providing persons with the information they want at the time they want it remains a challenge. Information must be tailored to individual literacy skills and meet their varying needs, as the experience and impact of osteoarthritis symptoms changes over time. In order to maximise the potential of persons to learn the required management skills and participate in decision-making, a web-based support tool will be developed based on the challenges and experiences that patients face (Brembo *et al.*, 2016). This tool is meant to provide its users with tailored evidence-based information and to serve as a self-evaluation tool by asking service users to keep track of their experiences, values, self-management strategies and symptoms over time. This track record aims to support the communication between the person and their healthcare professionals, to support self-management skills and to facilitate shared decision-making in clinical practice.

DEVELOPING TECHNOLOGY-SUPPORTED HEALTHCARE INTERVENTIONS IN A PERSON-CENTRED WAY

Healthcare services face major challenges in the future, partly due to demographic changes, including the steady increase of the ageing population and concomitant long-term conditions. To be able to handle these challenges, there is a need to develop effective models for restructuring health and care services, for allocation of resources and quality assurance of the service as well as the level and scope of competence. Every service user and their next of kin expects to be seen, heard and taken care of on a personalised, individual basis, regardless of the systems, levels or professionals they encounter. In a similar vein, the people working within the health and care services need a safe and efficient working environment in which they are both challenged and trusted. There is a need for both higher and broader (technological) competencies and a high degree of adaptability in order to meet future challenges.

In the western world, there is a parallel tendency to reallocate jobs and healthcare supply, from hospitals to primary and community care, from national or regional to local care services and between healthcare professions (e.g. practice nurses assuming doctors' tasks). The introduction of technology-based interventions and services and the consequent need for education, knowledge and new skills are important aspects in this on-going process. Although technology is not new to healthcare, the systematic utilisation of healthcare technology within all levels of healthcare demands a true paradigm shift in the delivery of health and care services and can thus be seen as an innovation in itself. A successful implementation of such innovations depends on the innovation itself, the health professional (individual), the organisation and the socio-political context (Fleuren *et al.*, 2014b). To achieve the pursued use and effectiveness it is, however, crucial to take into account the needs and demands of the individual end users in every step of the development process. A theoretical framework such as Intervention Mapping (IM) (Figure 13.1) or the Measurement Instrument for Determinants of Innovations (MIDI) may guide this development towards a person-centred intervention and guarantee an acceptable product and thereby successful implementation of the developed intervention (Bartholomew *et al.*, 2011; Fleuren *et al.*, 2014a; Van Bruinessen *et al.*, 2014). The IM framework systematically guides and documents the decisions through each step of the intervention development process. IM stresses the importance of developing theory and evidence-informed programmes taking an ecological approach to assessing and intervening on health problems and community participation. It incorporates theory and empirical evidence to identify determinants of behaviour, develop intervention objectives and select methods and strategies for an intervention (Bartholomew *et al.*, 2011).

The IM framework departs from needs assessment among the intended end users. This point of departure prevents the development of interventions that do not appeal to the target group; a feature well-known in the field of technology-driven interventions. The hip osteoarthritis

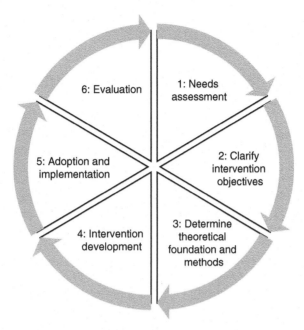

Figure 13.1 Modified version of the Intervention Mapping framework.

project, for instance, started with conducting interviews with individuals to find out what needs they had with regards to information and emotional support (Brembo *et al.*, 2016). The interviews revealed that persons with hip osteoarthritis are in great need of information and emotional support throughout the whole hip osteoarthritis continuum. Their needs, concerns and expectations must be appropriately understood and met by health providers caring for people living with hip osteoarthritis.

The knowledge and model developed through this study will be used as a basis for the development of a web-based tool for people living with hip osteoarthritis, their families and involved health providers, designed to increase service user knowledge and support communication during the process of preparing individualised care plans in clinical settings. The technology used in the digital night surveillance project has been developed by small and medium-sized technological enterprises based on the needs as defined by the management and employees in the health and care services of regional municipalities. The technology has been introduced (adopted) and then further developed (fine-tuned) during the implementation, in order to work optimally within each municipality. The researchers have been studying a range of the co-creation processes that have been ongoing during the phases of development and implementation: communication processes, learning processes, stakeholder analysis, service development processes and the processes from adoption to implementation and even continuation of the technology. The intervention developers used the MIDI as a quantitative measure of determinants relevant for healthcare professionals during the implementation process (*Fleuren et al.*, 2014a). The MIDI survey captures four categories of determinants:

1. The innovation.
2. The potential user of the innovation.
3. The organisation where the potential user works.
4. The socio-political context.

This survey is applied at different points in time throughout the implementation process with the purpose of evaluating the development and the impact of the innovation.

PRINCIPLES OF PERSON-CENTREDNESS GUIDING THE THREE PROJECTS

Each of the three technology-supported projects presented in this chapter has incorporated the principles of person-centredness in a different way. The web-based, self-management enhancing interventions for persons living with long-term conditions are person-centred in the sense that as part of these interventions, healthcare professionals provide personalised, situational feedback on a daily basis through smartphone or PDA, which is based on the input of the person. Service users complete online questionnaires in the form of an e-diary that reflects their current and often dysfunctional feelings, cognitions and activities. By receiving person-centred advice and suggestions, the service user's coping abilities can be strengthened and elaborated upon whereby self-management skills increase. An asset of the technology-supported interventions that furthermore strengthens the level of person-centredness is that the intervention is situational and knows no limits in terms of time and place; service users can choose their own time and manner for using the intervention. For the therapist, however, it remains a challenge to incorporate this, so far, time intensive intervention into their daily practice. The intervention seems therefore foremost person-centred for the service user, less so for the healthcare professional. The digital night surveillance of persons with dementia does seem to unburden the healthcare professional personally. Previously, the night shifts of the healthcare professional in dementia care meant being constantly alert to those residents who may wander, for example. The technology-supported preventive service takes away this demand and makes it possible to assist a resident before strong emotions and physical injury has occurred; the best of both worlds. The hip osteoarthritis project is person-centred in the way that the content of the future intervention will be guided by the input from those living with the condition as presented during the interviews at the needs assessment phase of the project. These needs guide the development and will be used as tailoring variables in the intervention, which makes the intervention more personally relevant in form and content.

KEY LEARNING

In this paragraph about lessons learned we look back at the three questions that guided this chapter:

1. *How can technology uplift today's healthcare services?* Clearly, technology can facilitate healthcare services in different ways. It can lighten the often-heavy burden of healthcare professionals' daily work and offer service users several facilities for use in their own time and place. As technology-supported interventions do ask for other expertise and experience, it so far remains a challenge to embed the use of these interventions within busy daily clinical practice. Besides, the use of technology-supported interventions does require specific expertise from the end user.
2. *Are technology-supported innovations person-centred?* The technology-supported interventions presented in this chapter each appear to be person-centred in their own way. This reflects the continuous evolution and broad operationalisation of the concept of

person-centredness; as long as a person (being the person of the service user or the person of the healthcare professional) benefits from an intervention which is adapted to his or her own experiences, needs or characteristics, the principles of person-centredness are safeguarded. Nevertheless, attention needs to be paid to the earlier-mentioned requirements for using technology-supported interventions. For each technology-supported intervention the question should be: is the person served by technology?

3. *How can technology enhance personhood?* Before technology met healthcare, numerous technology-supported interventions were developed because there was the technology to build them, not because end users needed them. Now the different fields have started working more closely together and the development process more often starts with a thorough needs assessment. Newly developed interventions become implemented and used more often and reach a wider public.

REFERENCES

Bartholomew, L.K., Parcel, G.S., Kok, G. *et al.* (2011) *Planning Health Promotion Programs: An Intervention Mapping Approach*, 3rd edition. Jossey-Bass, San Francisco.

Brembo, E.A., Kapstad, H., Eide, T. *et al.* (2016) Patient information and emotional needs across the hip osteoarthritis treatment and care continuum: a qualitative study. *BMC Health Services Research*, **16**, 88.

Craig, P., Dieppe, P., Macintyre, S. *et al.* (2008) Developing and evaluating complex interventions: the new Medical Research Council guidance. *BMJ*, **337**, a1655.

Fleuren, M.A., Paulussen, T.G., Van Dommelen, P. and Van Buuren, S. (2014a) Measurement Instrument for Determinants of Innovations (MIDI). https://www.tno.nl/media/6077/fleuren_et_al_midi_measurement_instrument.pdf (accessed 1 February 2017).

Fleuren, M.A., Paulussen, T.G., Van Dommelen, P. and Van Buuren, S. (2014b) Towards a measurement instrument for determinants of innovations. *International Journal for Quality in Health Care*, **26**, 501–510.

Krijgsman, J. and Klein Wolterink, J. (2012) Ordening in de wereld van eHealth *[Ordering in the world of eHealth] (whitepaper)*. Nictiz, Den Haag.

Kristjánsdóttir, O.B., Fors, E., Eide, E. *et al.* (2011) Written situational feedback via mobile phone to support self-management of chronic widespread pain: a usability study of a web based intervention. *BMC Musculoskeletal Disorders*, **12**, 51.

Kristjánsdóttir, O.B., Fors, E.A., Eide, E. *et al.* (2013a) A smartphone-based intervention with diaries and therapist-feedback to reduce catastrophizing and increase functioning in women with chronic widespread pain: randomized controlled trial. *Journal of Medical Internet Research*, **15**, e5.

Kristjánsdóttir, O.B., Fors, E.A., Eide, E. *et al.* (2013b) Smartphone-based diaries and therapist-feedback to promote self-management in women with chronic widespread pain following inpatient pain management program: 11-month follow-up results of a randomized trial. *Journal of Medical Internet Research*, **15**, e72.

Lai, C.K.Y. and Arthur, D.G. (2003) Wandering behaviour in people with dementia. *Journal of Advanced Nursing*, **44**, 173–182.

Murray, E. (2008) Internet-delivered treatments for long-term conditions: strategies, efficiency and cost-effectiveness. *Expert Review of Pharmacoeconomics and Outcomes Research*, **8**, 261–272.

Murray, E. (2009) The role of internet-delivered interventions in self-care, in *Shared Decision-Making in Health Care: Achieving Evidence-Based Patient Choice*, 2nd edition (eds A. Edwards and G. Elwyn). Oxford University Press, Oxford.

Nes, A., Dulmen, S. van, Eide, E. *et al.* (2012) The development and usability of a web-based intervention with diaries and situational feedback via smartphone to support self-management in patients with diabetes type 2. *Diabetes Research and Clinical Practice*, **3**, 385–393.

Nes, A.G., Eide, H., Kristjánsdóttir, O.B., Dulmen, S. van. (2013) Web-based, self-management enhancing interventions with e-diaries and personalized feedback for persons with chronic illness; a tale of three studies. *Patient Education and Counselling*, **93**, 451–458.

Nes, A.G., Brembo, E.A., Dulmen, S. van *et al.* (2014) Using acceptance and commitment therapeutical principles in a web-based intervention for women with chronic widespread pain – evaluating protocol adherence in text-based interventions. *International Journal of Person Centered Medicine*, **4**, 115–125.

Nilsen, E., Dugstad, J., Eide, H. *et al.* (2016) Exploring resistance to implementation of welfare technology in municipal healthcare services – a longitudinal case study. *BMC Health Services Research*, **16**, 657.

Oerlemans, S., Van Cranenburgh, O., Herremans, P.-J. *et al.* (2011) Intervening on cognitions and behaviour in irritable bowel syndrome: a feasibility trial using PDAs. *Journal of Psychosomatic Research*, **70**, 267–277.

Van Bruinessen, I.R., Weel-Baumgarten, E.M. van, Snippe, H.W. *et al.* (2014) User driven eHealth. Patient participatory development and testing of a computer tailored communication training for patients with malignant lymphoma. *Journal of Medical Internet Research Research Protocols*, **3**, e59.

Zhang, W., Moskowitz, R.W., Nuki, G. *et al.* (2008) OARSI recommendations for the management of hip and knee osteoarthritis, Part II: OARSI evidence-based, expert consensus guidelines. *Osteoarthritis and Cartilage/OARS, Osteoarthritis Research Society*, **16**, 137–162.

Editors' Commentary

There is little doubt that technology and healthcare go hand in hand and the use of technology permeates all aspects of healthcare practice. However, currently we are witnessing an unprecedented growth in the use of technology solutions for addressing health issues and practices, driven by economic and clinical effectiveness demands. Earlier in this book, Jacobs and colleagues (Chapter 5) made the case for the humanisation of ICT in healthcare and argued that 'Technology-supported healthcare can be humanising and dehumanising at the same time. When applying technology, it is important to consider and secure different aspects of person-centredness and regularly monitor end users' needs, experiences and perspectives'. Also in this book, Skovdahl and Dewing (Chapter 7) considered the ethical issues that arise when using technology in services for people living with dementia. All of these chapters make the same point explicit, i.e. that the use of technology in healthcare is not a simple solution, but brings with it a variety of complex issues that need to be thought through in order for the technology not to erode individual and collective personhood. Few of us would argue against advances that have been made in personalised medicine and robotics that have had significant impacts on tackling disease, increasing mortality rates, improving quality of life and making health services more efficient and effective. However, we have to be careful not to accept blindly technologies that can significantly erode individual autonomy, self-determination, freedom and human rights. Van Dulmen and colleagues illustrate these complexities through the three study examples presented – each one brings its own challenges in keeping personhood at the centre of decisions made and ensuring that the person does not become secondary to the 'testing' of the technology is a key challenge in each of the methodologies presented. Of course these challenges reflect the dynamic relationship that exists between person-centredness at the level of care delivery and the macro socio-political influences on this care delivery. ICT is big money and the lure of finding 'the solution' can overwhelm attention being paid to individual experience – although we are confident that the authors of this chapter are focused on the latter as a priority. The chapter does raise issues about methodologies used to test ICT solutions in healthcare and the need to ensure that these are person-centred also. Van Dulmen and colleagues illustrate the case made previously by Jacobs and colleagues (Chapter 5) that research into the testing of ICT solutions needs to adopt a mixed-methods approach incorporating innovative strategies for collaboration, participation and co-design. The language of 'end-user' continues to dominate this kind of research, so it is encouraging that van Dulmen challenges this discourse and propose ways for engaging key informants in all stages of the research. Of course, truly to advance this field of research, then it could be argued that healthcare researchers need to be much more radical and creative in their approaches and rather than merely adapting existing methodologies, they need to draw from designs outside of healthcare and particularly from the world of product design, creative industries and the arts. This is a key challenge to person-centred healthcare researchers of the future.

14 Learning to be an Effective Person-Centred Practitioner

Caroline Williams and Brendan McCormack

Reflective questions

1. What are the challenges in working with practitioners in a collaborative, inclusive and participative way, when most of them have been conditioned into a positivistic view of research and knowledge development?
2. What do you do to ensure you remain person-centred and facilitative, and avoid slipping into being paternalistic and overly supportive?
3. How do you ensure that the participants do not suddenly move from being participants in the study to being the objects of the study?
4. How do you reconcile working in research that in certain circles is not seen as 'legitimate' or 'high quality'?

OVERVIEW OF THE STUDY

Learning through work has the potential to develop both the individual practitioner and their practice in a way that classroom learning is unable to, but to achieve this the focus has to be in certain key areas, one of which is questioning existing ways of practice and challenging existing assumptions and cultures (Raelin, 2008). This is extremely difficult work, however, as it requires a practitioner to re-examine and shift some of their most fundamental beliefs; this can be extremely destabilising and the increased discomfort and anxiety not surprisingly causes most people to avoid it (Schein, 2004). Practitioners therefore need support to both identify and then question the everyday assumptions that underpin their practice and then further support to work through the resulting discomfort to change (Williams, 2010). It is this support that Rogers (1983) believes can be provided by a facilitator, developing learning from the student's own insight and experience, by assisting them to reflect critically. For practitioners who already assume their practice is person-centred, or who are working behind a self-protective façade, the challenge is to enable them to cast an analytical eye over their own practice, and most especially to help them to know themselves – one of the essential prerequisites in the person-centred practice framework (McCormack and McCance, 2017).

Person-Centred Healthcare Research, First Edition. Edited by Brendan McCormack, Sandra van Dulmen, Hilde Eide, Kirsti Skovdahl and Tom Eide.
© 2017 John Wiley & Sons Ltd. Published 2017 by John Wiley & Sons Ltd.

The aim of the study was to develop a detailed understanding of the role of the facilitator in enabling the development of nurses from a reflective appraisal system to engaging in critically reflective work-based learning. This chapter will focus on the methodology that is framing the study. It was developed specifically for this research and blends the Critical Companionship conceptual framework for facilitation (Titchen, 2000; Titchen, 2003) with constructs for a critical enquiry. The framework was developed through a process of critical creative inquiry using creative arts. Throughout the chapter we illustrate the elements of the framework using artistic and theoretical illustrations. The resultant Critical Companionship methodology is participative, action-oriented and transformational, with critical intent.

PRINCIPLES OF PERSON-CENTREDNESS GUIDING THE STUDY

The study is underpinned by three philosophical approaches: humanistic existentialism, hermeneutics and critical theory. The humanistic existentialist philosophical perspective holds that as persons we are unique individuals who actively participate in the world around us, making our own informed choices as we do so (Nyatanga and Dann, 2002). This means that we have the freedom to choose the sort of person that we are by the values we hold, the choices we make and the things that we do. It also follows from this that if we are all free to make of ourselves what we will, it is inconsistent to believe that one group of people are in some way superior or inferior to another group, as it assumes that people are predetermined to be something (Barnes, 1961). Humanistic existentialism is therefore completely opposed to the exploitation of others, and instead requires us to acknowledge the human dignity, freedom and integrity of other people, and to recognise what they need to enable them to realise their own freedom to choose (Greene, 1988). This is not suggesting that one person can somehow 'bestow' personhood on another, but rather it is a mutual recognition of each other's personhood. Freedom of choice, however, means that it is possible consciously to choose to treat someone with respect and dignity, or consciously to choose not to treat them that way. It is important therefore when making or acting on moral judgements about another person that we not only recognise that we are doing it, but also recognise our accountability and responsibility for that decision (Cooper, 1999; Sartre, 2007). It is this authentic way of being – ensuring that what we say and what we do are in alignment with our values and beliefs – that ultimately impacts on the way we develop and work with relationships that recognise the uniqueness of the other (Macmurray, 1961).

PROCESS AND OUTCOME EVALUATION

The above view of person-centredness directly influences not only the research methodology, but also the view of learning and the educational practices that are adopted within the study. The key principles for the study are therefore that: education and research should take place with people and not be something that is done to or for them; it should involve active, practical engagement with real experiences; it needs to be flexible to enable people the freedom and responsibility to make informed choices; and it should have a transformational intent, with an overall purpose of enabling people to reach their full potential and share in the generation of knowledge. To meet these principles the Critical

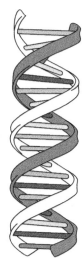

Companionship research methodology has developed as a double helix that contains both a learning strand and an enquiry strand. The methodology is represented in Figure 14.1 'unravelled' for ease of understanding.

The diagram illustrates the two strands of the double helix, where the learning strand contains the process concepts from Critical Companionship, and the enquiry strand contains the critical enquiry constructs (Figure 14.1). The framework is made up of four domains:

1. Being Person-Centred.
2. Being Intentional.
3. Being Facilitative.
4. Being Present.

In the following sections, the double helix diagram will be explained in detail. Each section is illustrated with a figure that is a representation of the relevant section derived from Figure 14.1.

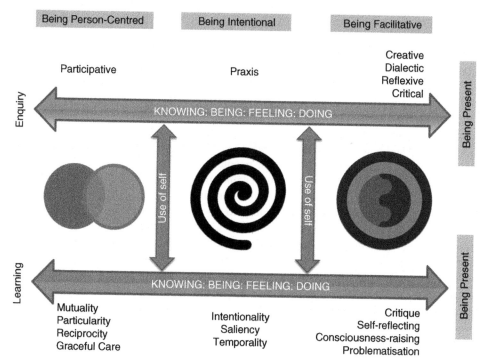

Figure 14.1   Diagrammatic representation of the Critical Companionship Methodology.

Being person-centred

Person-centredness developed from the work of Carl Rogers (1902–1987) and his approach to psychotherapy, and is concerned with being in a relationship with another person where the environment is one of unconditional positive regard, empathy and authenticity (Rogers, 1980). Similarly, Macmurray believes that we have three possible ways of relating to other

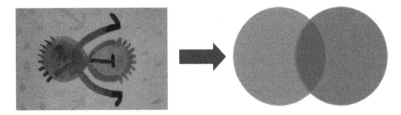

Figure 14.2 Creative development of the 'Being Person-Centred' domain.

people – an impersonal way, a functional way and a personal way. Each way of relating gives rise to a different knowledge of people (Macmurray, 1961), but it is only personal relationships that could be argued to be truly person-centred. Macmurray perceives 'friendship' as the deepest possible form of this personal relationship, where 'friendship' involves such things as mutuality, love, compassion, a focus on the other and sharing (Macmurray, 1961). 'Friendship' is therefore about equality and freedom, and highlights the importance of positive and ethical relationships between people, where acting ethically implies taking responsibility for our actions, and not doing things that will limit the freedom of others or prevent them from realising their goals. It is only in such a relationship that we can really relax and be ourselves, and the main reason for this is the trust between us.

In the 'Being Person-Centred' domain the learning strand is the relationship domain from Critical Companionship (Titchen, 2000; Titchen, 2003). This was developed from Campbell's theology of professional care (Campbell, 1984) and the work of Rogers (Rogers, 1983) and his helping relationship in an education context. It emphasises a carefully negotiated, non-hierarchical relationship where both parties share responsibility for learning (Titchen, 2000). The enquiry strand in the 'Being Person-Centred' domain considers the relationship between the researcher and practitioners that is needed to enable an appropriate investigation of the topic. It could be suggested that because the people in the study are the same (the facilitator/researcher and practitioners/participants), then once the relationship has been established for the learning strand (through the Relationship domain in Critical Companionship) then it would be impossible not to carry that through to the enquiry strand. However, Macmurray (1961) believes that, if required, it is possible to withdraw deliberately into an impersonal relationship and view the other person as an 'object'. The decision to remain in a personal relationship with the practitioners throughout the study was therefore an intentional one, befitting the philosophical stance. The construct in this enquiry strand is 'participative', where participative means something that is shared, and something that people are involved in. To that end the methodology works with the involvement of all parties in the creation of knowledge, and although we planned the structure of the study in advance, decisions made once the study was underway took place in collaboration with the practitioners, and some of the key features in the design of the methodology were there to make participation as easy as possible for the practitioners.

Being intentional

Existentialism as a philosophy emphasises the importance of action (Sartre, 2007), in that rather than having some predefined existence, people are what they do. To work with this therefore requires a methodology that is oriented toward action and transformation, enabling people to reach their full potential.

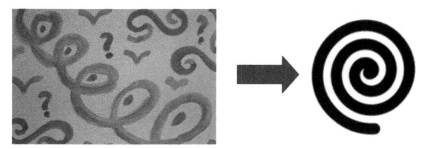

Figure 14.3 Creative development of the 'Being Intentional' domain.

In the 'Being Intentional' domain the learning strand is the 'Rationality-Intuitive' domain in Critical Companionship (Titchen, 2000). The three process concepts have both rational and intuitive dimensions, and are a combination of acting intentionally and with self-awareness, but also acting on intuition. In Critical Companionship this domain flows between the Relationship domain and the Facilitation domain, so that developing the relationship occurs at the same time as the facilitation. The enquiry strand in the 'Being Intentional' domain holds the construct Praxis. Praxis is an intentional process of thoughtful, mindful action, which is guided by a moral and ethical stance to act truly and justly (McCormack and Titchen, 2006). It is seen as an intertwined process, depicted by the spiral of constant movement, which has both a hermeneutic element and an emancipatory element (Titchen and McCormack, 2010). The hermeneutic element facilitates understanding and learning. The emancipatory element involves reflection to identify the constraints in a situation and enable action to be taken to overcome them. It is this constant intentional movement between understanding and action that brings about change. Change will not be achieved without practitioners increased understanding, but understanding alone will not automatically lead to change. In the methodology, it is the central positioning of the concept Praxis that turns the Critical Companionship conceptual framework for facilitation into a methodology for a critical enquiry that blends theory, practice and knowledge generation. Praxis is therefore the 'engine room' of the methodology, placed centrally and linked to all the other domains. It supports the critical intent of the study which is not only to develop knowledge, but also to bring about the emancipation and transformation of all participants.

Being facilitative

In the 'Being Facilitative' domain the learning strand is the Facilitation domain in Critical Companionship. This is concerned with raising awareness, supporting critical reflection, uncovering embedded knowledge and identifying potential areas for change (Titchen, 2000). It has an emancipatory cognitive interest (Habermas, 1987). The enquiry strand in the 'Being Facilitative' domain sets out the constructs that facilitate the generation of knowledge from the study. Critical research has three elements or movements (Alvesson and Deetz, 2000): an interpretative movement where participants' individual understandings of their experiences are captured and explored, producing insights into the issue being researched – facilitated in this methodology by using creative and dialectic processes; a reflexive movement where the things that impact on the understandings, and the insights and interpretations that are made from it, are identified; and a critical movement where alternative ways of thinking about, relating to, and changing what exists takes place. These three movements and four processes are blended with each other, being used as and when most appropriate to facilitate a deepening understanding:

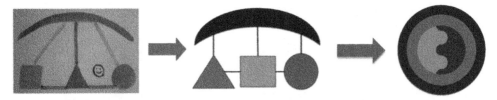

Figure 14.4 Creative development of the 'Being Facilitative' domain.

1. *Creative*. The creative arts were used both to support the development of the methodology, as well as being an integral part of it. Capturing something creatively is a form of presentational knowing and it is generally believed to emerge from, and be grounded in, experiential knowing (Heron and Reason, 1997). The time that it takes to create something is useful reflective time, and so using the creative arts can represent experiential knowing in richer, more expressive forms (Lliamputtong and Rumbold, 2008).

2. *Dialectic*. Dialectic refers to various methods of reasoning and open discussion, in which the key concepts are those of synthesis and change, and where parts are understood in relation to wholes. Dialectic thought therefore emphasises a 'both/and' position rather than an 'either/or' (Baxter and Montgomery, 1996, p. 6), and hence it enables multiple positions to be worked with, which is important when working with individuals in a group situation. In this study the whole dialectic process moves backwards and forwards between individual practitioners, their individual experiences and the group experiences; and between raw data and developing themes, using one to inform the other. By examining contradictions and complexities in this way a deeper understanding is developed.

   The creative and dialectic processes were integrated throughout the interpretative movement and were facilitated with the practitioners through a group process of Creative Reflective Analysis, which involved them interpreting, comparing and contrasting their own experience with that of others. We also engaged with creative and dialectic processes when comparing, contrasting and interpreting experiences during further analysis of data.

3. *Reflexive*. Reflexivity is a fluid process that is based on the idea of 'transforming personal experience into public and accountable knowledge' (Finlay, 2002, p. 533). The role of reflexivity is to highlight and explore the interdependence and connection between the researcher, the methodology and the data (Mauthner and Doucet, 2003). It involves questioning and exploring one's own assumptions and understandings (Freshwater and Rolfe, 2001) by engaging in explicit, self-aware analysis throughout the research process (Finlay, 2002, p. 536).

   The reflexive movement in the 'Being Facilitative' domain is approached from three angles and the resulting meta-analysis is used as additional data:

   - An introspective reflexive approach examining the impact of the researcher/critical companion on the study.
   - A relational reflexive approach examining the impact of the relationships in the study.
   - An epistemic reflexive approach examining the interpretation of data.

4. *Critical*. The critical movement of the 'Being Facilitative' domain works with the data that has resulted from the interpretative and reflexive movements above. The critical element aims to identify how and why the existing context constrains, influences and frustrates both the action and the interpretation of the participants, and suggests how to correct them.

These four processes (Creative, Dialectic, Reflexive, Critical) are blended and woven through different data collection and analysis methods so as to ensure coherence both with the philosophical stance and within the methodology.

Being present

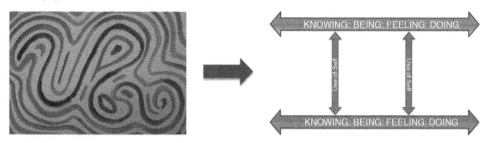

Figure 14.5   Creative development of the 'Being Present' domain.

One of the central tenets of existentialism is that living is participatory and involved, so any enquiry needs to acknowledge the importance of participation in the act of knowing (Macquarrie, 1972), and should therefore take place from an embedded position. It is the embedded nature of both the researcher and the practitioners that is highlighted in this domain.

The 'Being Present' domain is an overarching domain that is an extension of the 'Facilitative Use of Self' domain from Critical Companionship, which is identified as complex and dynamic, and involves the Critical Companion being able to use the other domains in the best mix to support the learning of the practitioner (Titchen, 2000). The 'Being Present' domain extends this to include the enquiry strand of the study, supporting and 'holding' the research. The domain contains the 'human' aspects 'doing, feeling, knowing and being', which represent the Critical Companion/researcher as a person, and also considers being aware of 'being in' and 'being with' the research, being authentic and embodying the process (McCormack, 2003).

STUDY PROGRESS

The macro design of the study was based around a cohort of practitioners as demonstrated in Figure 14.6 which illustrates one action cycle. There were two main action cycles that corresponded with the two periods of field work, each one lasting for a year. During each year of fieldwork each practitioner in the cohort was in an individual Critical Companionship relationship with Caroline (Titchen, 2000), which was planned to last one year and then formally end. To facilitate their learning the practitioners were working with Caroline as individuals, but in the enquiry process they were one of a group of participants. Each group met four times through the course of their year in the study, to analyse their data. Within the design there are therefore three main Praxis spirals:

1. The practitioners understanding and developing their own practice, facilitated by Caroline.
2. Caroline understanding and developing her own practice as a facilitator.
3. All of the participants as a group understanding and developing knowledge about the facilitation of work-based learning.

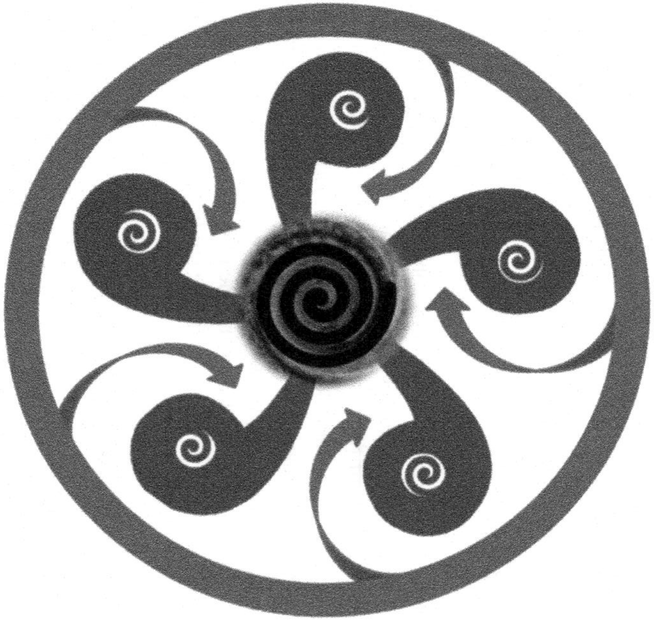

Symbol	Meaning
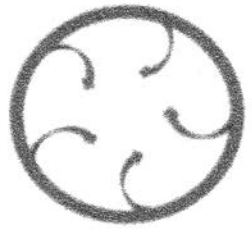	Caroline as the facilitator, acting as critical companion to five individual practitioners, facilitating the research, and 'holding' the study ('Being Present' domain)
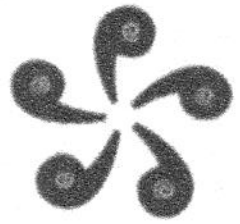	Five individual practitioners, working in a critical companionship relationship with Caroline, developing themselves and their practice individually through their own praxis spirals
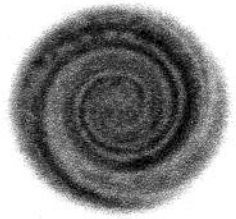	The coming together of all research participants (the practitioners and the researcher) to develop a deeper understanding of the mechanisms and processes necessary for the facilitation of learning through work; the constraints inherent in the culture and context of work; and how these can be transformed
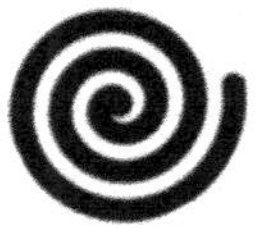	Caroline's praxis spiral as she reflexively explores her facilitation skills to come to a greater understanding, and to transform her practice to make her more effective

Figure 14.6 The research operational framework.

CONCLUSION

At the time of writing this chapter, the fieldwork for the study had been completed and data from the study are still being analysed. For the participants in the study learning to be effective person-centred practitioners has been challenging. One of the practitioners summed up her change in an email to Caroline:

> *[...] I thought I was a reflective practitioner before.... I would think how things made me feel, my colleagues, my patients and to some degree would think how I could have improved on a situation. But now, I'm more person-centred. I think while I'm doing. I think about the service I'm giving. What is really important to the patients, to me. I want to feel like I'm a good nurse and what I'm doing is the best I can offer. I've upped my game. I think about the whole picture with the patient in the middle. It's so hard to pin point what's changed in me. I wasn't an unthinking nurse in the first place [but] I really do think that being 'heard' by you has made me feel valuable, that what I think and feel is important. When a person feels like that, they can grow. [...]. Emma*

KEY LEARNING

The key learning from undertaking this research has distilled into two main areas:

1. The importance of authenticity throughout the research. There is a requirement to develop a good understanding of the underpinning philosophical position and one's own values and beliefs in relation to this. This is needed to justify the choice of methodology as well as ensure coherence across the study, both during the planning phase as well as the operational phase. As a novice person-centred researcher, Caroline was helped to maintain this authentic stance by a good support structure of expert person-centred researchers.
2. The importance of the positioning of the participants in the study. When most practitioners have been conditioned into a positivistic view of research and knowledge development it is difficult to work with them in a collaborative, inclusive and participative way. The practitioners are expecting to be researched *on* rather than researched *with* and they can take some time to move from seeing themselves as 'guinea pigs', to being able and willing to participate in knowledge generation. There are also challenges when undertaking data analysis to ensure that the practitioners remain as people, and do not degenerate into becoming objects within the study. This was achieved by ensuring that the data were not divorced from the practitioners, and that their words were not analysed in isolation from them as people. Data were therefore interpreted using a hermeneutic approach, constantly moving from the individual's data to the data generated by the group, keeping data together and ensuring that all extracts were kept connected to their context.

The implications for person-centred research from these key learning points are the importance of ensuring that the person-centred stance is made explicit at the outset of the research and that all aspects of the study are then congruent with that. They also point to the need for collaborative working between experts in the field to illustrate person-centred principles in action; to provide critical challenge to enable authenticity; and to ensure support for novice person-centred researchers.

REFERENCES

Alvesson, M. and Deetz, S. (2000) *Doing Critical Management Research*. Sage, London.

Barnes, H. (1961) *The Literature of Possibility. A Study in Humanistic Existentialism*. Tavistock Publications, London.

Baxter, L.A. and Montgomery, B.M. (1996) *Dialogues and Dialectics*. The Guilford Press, New York.

Campbell, A.V. (1984) *Moderated Love*. SPCK, London.

Cooper, D.E. (1999) *Existentialism: A Reconstruction*, 2nd edition. Blackwell Publishing, Oxford.

Finlay, L. (2002) 'Outing' the researcher: the provenance, process and practice of reflexivity. *Qualitative Health Research*, **12**, 531–545.

Freshwater, D. and Rolfe, G. (2001) Critical reflexivity: a politically and ethically engaged research method for nursing. *Journal of Research in Nursing*, **6**, 526–537.

Greene, M. (1988) *The Dialectic of Freedom*. Teacher's College Press, New York.

Habermas, J. (1987) Appendix: knowledge and human interests: a general perspective, in *Knowledge and Human Interest*, 2nd edition (ed. J. Habermas). Polity Press, Cambridge. pp. 301–317.

Heron, J. and Reason, P. (1997) A participatory inquiry paradigm. *Qualitative Inquiry*, **3**, 274–294.

Lliamputtong, P. and Rumbold, J. (2008) Knowing differently: setting the scene, in *Knowing Differently: Arts-based and Collaborative Research Methods* (eds P. Lliamputtong and J. Rumbold). Nova Science Publishers, New York. pp. 1–23.

McCormack, B. (2003) Researching nursing practice: does person-centredness matter? *Nursing Philosophy*, **4**, 179–188.

McCormack, B. and McCance, T. (2017) *Person-Centred Practice in Nursing and Health Care: Theory and Practice*. Wiley Blackwell, Oxford.

McCormack, B. and Titchen, A. (2006) Critical creativity: melding, exploding, blending. *Educational Action Research*, **14**, 239–266.

Macmurray, J. (1961) *Persons in Relation*. Humanity Books, New York.

Macquarrie, J. (1972) *Existentialism*. Pelican Books, Harmondsworth.

Mauthner, N.S. and Doucet, A. (2003) Reflexive accounts and accounts of reflexivity in qualitative data analysis. *Sociology*, **37**, 413–431.

Nyatanga, L. and Dann, K.L. (2002) Empowerment in nursing: the role of philosophical and psychological factors. *Nursing Philosophy*, **3**, 234–239.

Raelin, J.A. (2008) *Work-Based Learning*. Jossey-Bass, San Francisco.

Rogers, C. (1980) *A Way of Being*. Houghton Mifflin Company, Boston.

Rogers, C. (1983) *Freedom to Learn for the 80s*. Charles E. Merrill, London.

Sartre, J. (2007) *Existentialism and Humanism*. Methuen & Co., London.

Schein, E.H. (2004) *Organizational Culture and Leadership*, 3rd edition. Jossey-Bass, San Francisco.

Titchen, A. (2000) *Professional Craft Knowledge in Patient-Centred Nursing and the Facilitation of its Development*. Ashdale Press, Kidlington.

Titchen, A. (2003) Critical companionship: part 1. *Nursing Standard*, **18**, 33–40.

Titchen, A. and McCormack, B. (2010) Dancing with stones: critical creativity as a methodology for human flourishing. *Educational Action Research*, **18**, 531–554.

Williams, C. (2010) Understanding the essential elements of work-based learning and its relevance to everyday clinical practice. *Journal of Nursing Managment*, **18**, 624–632.

Editors' Commentary

Some of the origins of person-centredness can be traced back to the work of Carl Rogers and his focus on humanistic principles in counselling and in the facilitation of learning. Rogers was particularly focused on 'the person' in learning situations and how person-hood should act as the 'rudder' for engaging in significant learning. Rogers also saw learning as a reciprocal process between co-learners, freeing learners from a subjugated relationship with 'teachers'. Instead both teacher and learner are in a co-learning relationship underpinned by humanistic relational principles geared towards transformation. Much has been written about 'creating freedom to learn' and how best to do this, but yet, the majority of curricula in healthcare professional education continue to be dominated by a teacher-led view of what needs to be learned and content that is often pre-prescribed with little space for individual choice about learning. While there are examples of curricula that aim to challenge this dominant learning paradigm, it continues to be the case that these are 'examplers' rather than a norm. The research being undertaken in this chapter, while incredibly complex, is a solid attempt at generating a truly person-centred approach to facilitating learning. It is no surprise to us that the methodology developed is complex as it demonstrates the complexity of the challenge that theorists such as Rogers and others pose if we are to genuinely engage with transformational learning. The processes of engagement that the authors outline require a high level of facilitation knowledge, skill and expertise and there lies the 'rub'. While the essence of the methodology being worked with is that of co-learning and authentic engagement, the reality is that facilitation of the process (which includes an integrated research/evaluation process) requires at least one partner in the relationship to have this advanced facilitation expertise. So can the relationship be really equal in this situation? One way of answering this question is to focus on what each person brings to the relationship as 'authentic persons'. While this may mean different levels of knowledge, skills and expertise, a willingness by all parties to suspend 'ego' in this situation and instead focus on what the philosopher Jacques Derrida saw as the gift of knowledge exchange that happens through deconstruction of experience. The elements of the framework presented in this chapter help this deconstruction to happen in a systematic way and in a way that respects the personhood of the 'other'. But as the authors rightly acknowledge, it cannot be assumed that those entering such a learning situation are 'ready' for the engagement needed. From childhood, we are socialised into a form of learning that is largely positivistic in nature with a focus on facts and outcomes. Transformational learning requires such a focus to be 'let go' in order for new possibilities to be 'let come' – a vessel that is already full cannot hold more liquid! We need to be able to let go of existing presuppositions and assumptions in order for new learning to arise and the potential for transformation to be realised. Clearly the framework presented in this chapter has much work to be done in testing it out in a variety of contexts in order to make it usable in a variety of learning situations. However as an approach to person-centred learning, including an integrated approach to the evaluation of that learning, it holds much potential.

15 Doing Eye and Vision Research in a Person-Centred Way

Rigmor C. Baraas, Lene A. Hagen, Hilde R. Pedersen and Jon V.B. Gjelle

---

Reflective questions

1. Being the healthcare professional: consider making a decision about treatment of an individual person according to results from a population-based study. What are the limitations?
2. Being the healthcare leader: consider making decisions on a health system level according to results based on one or a few persons. What are the limitations?
3. Being the person who needs healthcare: consider the implications if you are to make decisions about your own vision and eye health and/or choices about your own treatment based on (1) versus (2).

INTRODUCTION

The goal of person-centred eye and vision research is similar to that of other kinds of person-centred research. It is to describe, predict, explain and understand how each of us perceives the world – literally – through one's own eyes. It is to understand basic mechanisms of eye care, why things go wrong and how to prevent this, whether vision treatment or rehabilitation is needed and to develop and validate new ways of treatment. This knowledge will improve the outcomes of vision and eye health for each of us. Why? Because, one's vision and eye health are important predictors of how well we do at school, in daily life, at work and in one's spare time (World Health Organization, 2010). It is an important predictor of how well each of us will be able to cope on our own when we grow old (Paul and Yuanlong, 2012). Good vision and eye health are, in other words, important in all parts of life.

Person-Centred Healthcare Research, First Edition. Edited by Brendan McCormack, Sandra van Dulmen, Hilde Eide, Kirsti Skovdahl and Tom Eide.

OVERVIEW OF EYE AND VISION RESEARCH IN A PERSON-CENTRED CONTEXT

Vision is a subjective experience, based on inputs of photons of light that enter the eye. The physical properties of the light that bounces off the objects you observe are as important as the physical parameters of the eye when it comes to what kind of visual experience you have (as opposed to the person next to you). The light rays may or may not come to focus at the back of the eye. Photons are to a greater or lesser extent absorbed by the eye's photoreceptor cells, depending on what pigments these contain. These cells will transform the absorbed photons to signals that are conveyed to the brain, and this will create your personal visual experience. (For an introduction to the basics of vision, see Snowden, Thompson and Troscianko, 2012.)

Eye and vision research and its intended outcome are primarily geared towards increasing knowledge to help individuals with a vision problem. There is a good tradition for examining a few individuals very thoroughly, even describing the differences between them or describing individual changes over a period of months and years. For example, our group has been working on understanding vision in people who have a tritan colour vision deficiency caused by a specific genetic mutation (Baraas *et al.*, 2012) and how their vision changes over the course of a few years (Hagen *et al.*, 2015a). We have also been looking at structural changes in the eye of young adults, changes that may be important in terms of understanding who will develop age-related changes that may cause loss of vision. However, there is no tradition for describing eye and vision research in a person-centred context. The case example presented in Box 15.1 reflects this, and the aim was to see if methodology explicitly described as person-centred in psychopathology research can be useful for eye and vision research.

PRINCIPLES OF PERSON-CENTREDNESS GUIDING THE RESEARCH

An overarching principle of person-centred research involves respect for the individual person, their individual experiences, perceptions and preferences. These values influence the purpose and the process of research and affect how we recruit, engage and communicate with the participants and collect data.

There is large inter-individual variability in how each of us perceives the world around us (e.g. Dees *et al.*, 2015), because of the variability in physical parameters of the different structures of the eye (e.g. Dees *et al.*, 2011) and the large diversity in the genetic makeup of these structures (e.g. pigments in retinal photoreceptor cells, see Neitz and Neitz, 2011). There is a large intra-individual variability in how vision develops and changes as we grow and age (e.g. Spear, 1993). Understanding this variability and perhaps most importantly, variability in various combinations of parameters, is essential if we are to understand vision in general. This is also essential if we are to understand who will grow up with or without vision problems during teenage years or who will have good or bad vision and eye health when entering their older years (90+).

For the sake of argument, let us consider refractive errors. There is a combination of parameters that together make some people see the world around them in focus without any blur. Others have variations of these parameters that make the world around them blurry, and they need glasses or contact lenses to correct the refractive error to be able to see the world

Box 15.1   A case of tritan colour-vision deficiency

A young woman arrives at the lab for participation in a research project. She has signed up for participation because she is curious about her own colour vision. A qualitative interview with a few guiding questions about her vision and health is conducted after going through the written information about the research. During this interview, the woman describes problems with distinguishing the blue and green tokens of the Ludo board game when the light levels are a little low. That is, there is enough light for everyone else to see the difference in colour between the tokens, but she herself is having great difficulties and finds it hard to play the game. She finds it puzzling as she never experiences any problems distinguishing these colours when the light levels are higher. We carry out standard tests of colour vision under standard conditions. She behaves as if she has normal colour vision under these conditions. This makes us very curious, and we decide that we need to design an experiment to try to understand this. This is an experiment whereby her colour vision is tested under different levels of light, and both under dark adapted and light adapted conditions. The latter is necessary in terms of understanding whether the sensory cells that work during the night (rod cells) play a role in her colour perception when she experiences difficulties. It turns out that when light levels are low she behaves as if she has no blue (short-wavelength sensitive) cones. This colour vision deficiency is termed tritan deficiency. Cones are the sensory cells that work during daylight and that are important for perceiving colours and discriminating details (such as letters for reading). This leads us to investigate several members of her family with the same experiment and to carry out genetic analyses of the gene code for the short-wavelength sensitive pigment that resides in cones. She and the other members of her family whom all behaved as tritans had the same novel mutation – causing the blue cones to not function properly when the light levels are low (Baraas *et al.*, 2012). The person-oriented approach when enrolling participants affects how we recruit, engage and communicate with the participants, and is essential to understand better each person's individual visual experience. It ensures mutual understanding of why the research being carried out is needed. It empowers the individual through a better understanding of their own visual function. In this case it also led us to frame a problem that gave us new and novel insight about colour perception.

in focus. We have gained a lot of knowledge about vision over the last 40 years, but we still do not understand why some people become short-sighted and why others become long-sighted. Similarly, we still do not know why some people get age-related changes in their 50s whereas others reach 90 years old before loss of vision impacts on independence and daily living activities to any degree. The large inter-individual variability in vision can be observed in young persons, and we observe that the variability decreases with increasing age when only individuals who are considered to have normal healthy eyes are included in the study (Dees *et al.*, 2015). However, we do not know which combinations of parameters are of importance for preserving good vision and eye health as we age. There is so far little knowledge about intra-individual variability as we grow up and grow older. Importantly, studying just one parameter on its own is not enough. Some parameters are more important than others and the key is to understand which combinations and what parameters play a role. This will help us predict the outcome of vision and eye health for individual persons.

Let us continue with the refractive error example. How do we find the parameters and combinations that are important for understanding who will develop short-sightedness and who will develop long-sightedness? Eye and vision research can adopt different methodologies to address this question and a combination of observational and experimental studies may be needed. Eye and vision research quite often involves quantitative measures of optical and anatomical structures as well as physiological and perceptual function. This does not mean that qualitative measures are not included. A quantitative study may originate from a qualitative approach. A research question may arise from a description of a phenomenon made by a person with a particular visual experience or a vision problem. To build understanding for how this person uses their vision and what they do to circumvent the described problem, a qualitative interview with a few guiding questions may be useful. Through such an interview, it is sometimes possible to build enough knowledge to frame the basics of the problem and identify valid research questions. This will guide what measures are needed to be able to discuss the research questions asked.

For example, we may need to find out if the development of refractive errors is related to the degree in which the world is perceived as blurry. This may involve designing a new psychophysical measure to test perceptions of blur, unless we already have a method at hand. A new psychophysical experiment requires a series of pilot experiments before arriving at a valid one. This is an essential step and validation requires the use of standard quantitative analyses. As well as a measure of visual perceptual function, an electrophysiological experiment to measure electrical activity in the eye or in the brain may be included. The aim of such experiments is to find a mathematical description of the functional relationship between variations in the physical properties of the visual stimuli and the resulting variation in visual perception (Macmillan and Creelman, 2004). It is also necessary to measure parameters of the structures of the eye and possibly analyse the gene code for the pigments in the photoreceptor cells. The measures of the eye will tell us about the type and degree of refractive error and will give us the dimensions of the parts that contribute to focusing light at the back of the eye (Schwartz, 2013). The gene code can tell us about the properties of the pigments and to what extent each person's photoreceptor cells absorb the light in the visual stimuli (Dees *et al.*, 2011; Hofmann and Palczewski, 2015).

Person-centred eye and vision research requires a combination of measures that lend themselves to be modelled in a sensible manner. This has been described as to find 'the pattern of indivisible factors' (Bergman and Wangby, 2014). That is, the aim is to create a systematic view of biological and psychological parameters and analyse their associations with, for example, different types and degrees of refractive errors – to see beyond bits and pieces. To see each person as 'an organised whole with elements operating together to achieve a functioning system in a dynamic process with interactions between components', is termed 'the holistic-interactionistic research paradigm' (Magnusson, 1988; Magnusson and Törestad, 1993). Sterba and Bauer (2010) listed six principles and four methods for analysing a model-based person-oriented approach for psychopathology research. Here, we will *reflect* on whether these may also be the underpinnings for person-centred eye and vision research.

The six principles are:

1. *Individual specificity.* The eye and visual process is unique to each person.
2. *Complex interactions.* Vision is a biological–psychological–physical system, a cosmos of dynamic neural structures and processes that interact.
3. *Inter-individual differences in intra-individual change.* It is expected that vision and the eye will change as we grow and age, and that it will be in a predictable and structured manner, at least in healthy and normal development and ageing.

4. *Pattern summary*. It is expected that vision develops in a predictable way that can be described as patterns of the involved factors, but individuals or groups of individuals that may share the same pattern have not been studied over time.
5. *Holism*. The meaning of the involved factors is determined by the interactions among these factors.
6. *Pattern parsimony*. Even if patterns of the involved factors in vision development are somewhat unexplored (see principle 4), it is expected that there will be few patterns that are more frequently encountered than others.

The four statistical methods for analyses associated with the six principles according to Sterba and Bauer (2010) are:

- Less restrictive variable oriented methods (latent growth curve modelling) (principles 1, 2, 3 and 5).
- Classification (latent class growth) (principles 2 and 6).
- Hybrid classification (growth modelling) (principles 1–6).
- Single subject (dynamic factor analyses) (principles 1, 3, 4, 5, 6).

The principles that eye and vision research has a lot to gain from are: (2) complex interactions (from variations in the physical properties of the visual stimuli, to parameters of the eye, and the resulting variation in visual perception); (3) inter-individual differences in intra-individual change; and (4) pattern summary (is there a particular set of parameters of the eye that lead to a particular type of perception that is more common than other patterns?). Some work will gain momentum from the basis of standard quantitative analyses, but the statistical method that may influence future work is classification, that will allow grouping of longitudinal data according to trajectory groups (Nagin and Odgers, 2010), for example, to try to understand the differences in the trajectories of how refractive errors develop in different populations.

PROCESS AND OUTCOME EVALUATION

There are lessons to be learned from studying both inter- versus intra-individual variability. The research question needs to be explored to find what approach is most appropriate. Even if the final goal of person-centred research is knowledge at the level of the individual person, it may not be possible to answer the research question with one approach. Let us say that our main concern is to understand how refractive errors change as we grow up and grow older. What do we know? Is there a need to build an understanding of inter-individual variation at a given time point for individuals at different ages? Is there hetero- or homogeneity at each age? If a great deal of data has been reported previously, a systematic review of published data is needed. If not, a study looking at inter-individual variation might be the first step. Both will guide us to the age we might consider as a good starting point for performing a follow-up study on a smaller group of individuals and what method to choose. The choice of method must be weighed against the risk of drawing a false conclusion about one person from the mean of the population (ecological fallacy) versus drawing a false conclusion about aggregated data based on data from one or a few persons (atomistic fallacy) (Sterba and Bauer, 2010). The question that arises is whether we can use the results to generalise to a population and from this build an understanding of how to treat a random individual person. Molenaar (2015) argued that subject-specific methods are the most robust allowing for empirical evaluation of participant-specific principles rather than a priori assumptions. However, this is a method that may also require measures of many variables at several time points, thus asking the participant for substantial devotion to a particular project.

An interesting aspect is the conjectured differences in the trajectories of how refractive errors develop in populations with differences in the genes that code the photoreceptor pigments, such as for example Northern people as compared with Southeast Asians (Davidoff, 2015). The onset of short-sightedness is much earlier in Southeast Asians with a frequency around 10% in 7-year-olds, over 40% in 12-year-olds and over 70% in 18-year-olds (Dirani et al., 2009; Jin et al., 2015). In comparison, the frequency of short-sightedness is less than 20% in 17-year-old Northern people (Hagen et al., 2015b). This may not be related to the total time spent outdoors, but rather a combination of genetics, other biological factors and perhaps the temporal aspects of time spent outdoors during ordinary school days from a young age. It would be useful to perform longitudinal studies on both groups to understand differences in developmental and behavioural factors that play a role in the growth of the eye. Thus, a person-centred approach may help us understand what we have to do at what age level to combat the epidemic of short-sightedness in Southeast Asia.

KEY FINDINGS AND IMPACTS ON PERSONS, PEOPLE AND POPULATIONS

A person-centred approach can be applied to identify individuals and/or subpopulations of individuals who share similar characteristics of how their eyes and vision develop and mature. Knowledge from eye and vision research will have an impact on person-centred vision care, both in terms of *for* and *with* the person. Building knowledge about eye and visual function in subpopulations will help the eye healthcare professional to increase competence for communication about symptoms and needs, thereby facilitating early diagnosis as well as treatment and a successful outcome. This will help persons with a vision problem by building knowledge about their vision, and how they can take care of their own eyes and vision health. In other words, this can help the person become more empowered.

REFLECTIONS ON DOING PERSON-CENTRED RESEARCH AND BEING A PERSON-CENTRED RESEARCHER

The components addressed in this chapter (behavioural and biological factors, and environmental factors) may also be important with regards to understanding vision and eye health. Vision comes about because of processes in a biological system, and there is nothing contradictory between a natural science view of how to understand a dynamic system compared with a person-centred view (Magnusson, 1988). The aim is to understand how components operate and interact to achieve a functioning visual system in relation to the individual person's challenges, needs and values. The research should improve the outcome of vision and eye health for each person through understanding the many parts that form the organised whole that makes each a visual behaving person. But will our research lead to personalised vision care? Yes, but not in the sense that the person doesn't make an informed choice. It is necessary to consider treatment options for conditions (that may not be a disease) with an aim to improve visual function, and this involves mutual understanding of the problem and the person's needs. This requires that the interaction between participants and researchers is based on good communication and mutual trust in order to understand the person's abilities, needs and interests. Treatment today may be to optimise the person's vision and eye health, so any form of vision or eye problem will not hinder one's development and/or potential. That is, the short-term goal of treatment is to maintain or improve quality of life. Treatment in the long term may be to prevent development of vision problems, eye disease, illness, injury or any physical or mental impairment to improve long-term prospects of quality of life.

Early intervention is sometimes crucial to ensure quality of life in the long term, but it is also important to reflect on the consequence of informed choice of treatment as early as possible – the burden of knowledge about self.

KEY LEARNING

Person-centred eye and vision research requires a biological system view and quantitative analyses. In addition, we need to understand the differences between inter- and intra-individual variation and the appropriateness of choice of methods. Further, a key issue identified in this chapter is that of the need to understand the implications of ecological versus atomistic fallacy.

REFERENCES

Baraas, R.C., Hagen, L.A., Dees, E.W. and Neitz, M. (2012) Substitution of isoleucine for threonine at position 190 of S-opsin causes S-cone-function abnormalities. *Vision Research*, **73**, 1–9.

Bergman, L.R. and Wangby, M. (2014) The person-oriented approach: a short theoretical and practical guide. *Eesti Haridusteaduste Ajakiri*, **2**, 29–49.

Davidoff, C. (2015) *Cone Opsin Gene Variants in Color Blindness And Other Vision Disorders.* PhD thesis. University of Washington, Seattle, USA. https://dlib.lib.washington.edu/researchworks/bitstream/handle/1773/33578/Davidoff_washington_0250E_15133.pdf?sequence=1andisAllowed=y (accessed 1 February 2017).

Dees, E.W., Dubra, A. and Baraas, R.C. (2011) Variability in parafoveal cone mosaic in normal trichromatic individuals. *Biomedical Optics Express*, **2**, 1351–1358.

Dees, E.W., Gilson, S.J., Neitz, M. and Baraas, R.C. (2015) The influence of L-opsin gene polymorphisms and neural ageing on spatio-chromatic contrast sensitivity in 20-71 year olds. *Vision Research*, **116**, 13–24.

Dirani, M., Tong, L., Gazzard, G. *et al.* (2009) Outdoor activity and myopia in Singapore teenage children. *British Journal of Ophthalmology*, **93**, 997–1000.

Hagen, L.A., Gilson, S.J. and Baraas, R.C. (2015). Six-year follow-up of individuals heterozygous for the T190I mutation in the S-cone-opsin gene (OPN1SW). *Investigative Ophthalmology and Visual Science*, **56**, 4015.

Hagen, L.A., Gjelle, J.V.B., Arnegard, S. *et al.* (2015) Prevalence of refractive errors and colour vision deficiencies among Norwegian high school students. *Scandinavian Journal of Optometry and Visual Science*, **8**, 1–2.

Hofmann, L. and Palczewski, K. (2015) Advances in understanding the molecular basis of the first steps in color vision. *Progress in Retinal and Eye Research*, **49**, 46–66.

Jin, J-X., Hua, W-J., Jiang, X. *et al.* (2015) Effect of outdoor activity on myopia onset and progression in school-aged children in northeast China: the Sujiatun eye care study. *BMC Ophthalmology*, **15**, 73.

Macmillan, N.A. and Creelman, C.D. (2004) *Detection Theory: A User's Guide*, 2nd edition. Psychology Press, Hove.

Magnusson, D. (1988) *Individual Development from an Interactional Perspective: A Longitudinal Study.* Lawrence Erlbaum Associates, Hillsdale.

Magnusson, D. and Törestad, B. (1993) A holistic view of personality: a model revisited. *Annual Review of Psychology*, **44**, 427–452.

Molenaar, P.C.M. (2015) On the relation between person-oriented and subject-specific approaches. *Journal of Person Oriented Research*, **1**, 34–41.

Nagin, D.S. and Odgers, C.L. (2010) Group-based trajectory modeling (nearly) two decades later. *Journal of Quantitative Criminology*, **26**, 445–453.

Neitz, J. and Neitz, M. (2011) The genetics of normal and defective color vision. *Vision Research*, **51**, 633–651.

Paul, S. and Yuanlong, L. (2012) Inadequate light levels and their effect on falls and daily activities of community dwelling older adults: a review of literature. *New Zealand Journal of Occupational Therapy*, **59**, 39–42.

Schwartz, S. (2013) *Geometrical and Visual Optics*, 2nd edition. McGraw-Hill Education, London.

Snowden, R., Thompson, P. and Troscianko, T. (2012) *Basic Vision: An Introduction to Visual Perception*, 2nd edition. Oxford University Press, Oxford.

Spear, P.D. (1993) Neural bases of visual deficits during aging. *Vision Research*, **33**, 2589–2609.

Sterba, S.K. and Bauer, D.J. (2010) Matching method with theory in person oriented developmental psychopathology research. *Developmental Psychopathology*, **22**, 239–25.

World Health Organization (2010) *Action Plan for the Prevention of Avoidable Blindness and Visual Impairment, 2009–2013*. WHO Press, Geneva.

Editors' Commentary

In this book so far, readers might be forgiven for thinking that person-centred research focuses primarily on qualitative and participatory methodologies. So this chapter by Baraas and colleagues acts as an appropriate 'jolt' to that thinking! The chapter addresses an area of research that is in essence a highly scientific endeavour where the focus is on diagnosis and treatment. However, if we stop and think about vision health as an exemplar of many health issues, then it acts as an appropriate point of reflection regarding how we can make healthcare more person-centred. The authors of the chapter make a clear case for an individualised approach to vision health and of course many of the reasons why a person-centred approach is important in this field of practice also apply to many other aspects of health. However, what is important here is that while the arguments for individualised and person-centred healthcare are well played out in the literature, there is little evidence of research methods carrying through this same kind of thinking. Baraas and colleagues articulate principles for a person-centred approach to vision health research and these are easily applicable across other areas of research. The need to not always particularise from the general and vice versa is a powerful argument for more development of person-centred research approaches and this is a challenge for many areas of health research. As the authors highlight, this is not a case of interfering with the need for appropriately powered large studies that are generalisable. But it does make the case for carefully and systematically researching at the individual level, and as well as planning appropriate treatments to meet the individual needs arising, to also use these findings to inform generalisable studies. The authors also demonstrate ways in which qualitative and quantitative data collection methods can complement each other, not in a mixed-methods mode of practice, but as sequential stages in the planning of a series of questions over time – all of which ultimately inform the development of more person-centred practices as well as operationalising a person-centred programme of research. The chapter as a whole acts as an exemplar for such research developments and the work deserves to be seen in this context by other researchers who may be struggling to understand how their research could adopt more of a person-centred approach.

16 Person-Centred Communication Research: Systematic Observation of Real Life Practice

Hilde Eide, Linda Hafskjold, Vibeke Sundling and Sandra van Dulmen

---

Reflective questions

1. What is person-centred communication?
2. What roles do cues and concerns play in person-centred communication research?
3. How can person-centred communication research contribute to person-centred care?

INTRODUCTION

Communication is a cornerstone of healthcare – connecting service user and provider, building the relationship, and exchanging information and advice (Eide and Eide, 2007). Person-centred communication enables the expression of experiences, thoughts and ideas by service users and makes it possible for the healthcare provider to adapt the communication to the person's emotional and information needs. The etymological roots of the word communication are the Latin words, 'communis' and 'communicare'. Communis is a noun, which means common, communality or sharing. Whereas, communicare is a verb, which means 'make something common'. These meanings, common and sharing, open up for a broad research area within person-centred healthcare research.

In this chapter we will focus on one methodology for doing person-centred communication research, i.e. observational research into everyday healthcare practice. The international comparative research project that illustrates this method is set within the field of home care (Hafskjold *et al.*, 2015). The study aims to capture the communication practices and the challenges met in home care, as well as to look for examples of best practices. More specifically, the study focuses on service users' communication of concerns and worries and how nurses and nurse assistants respond to these utterances (Hafskjold *et al.*, 2016; Sundler *et al.*, 2016).

Observing behaviour in the context where it occurs is a basic human skill, linked both to evolutionary survival processes and to everyday social and relational life. Observational research can be traced from a naturalistic paradigm in social sciences, but the observer

---

Person-Centred Healthcare Research, First Edition. Edited by Brendan McCormack, Sandra van Dulmen, Hilde Eide, Kirsti Skovdahl and Tom Eide.

includes an interpretive position, given that human action always is infused with meaning. Therefore, the methodological point of departure for modern communication research is ethnography, where audio and video recordings as well as text-based material are the windows into people's interactions.

Communication research is inherently a qualitative process, as interpretation is basic to all communication research. The methodology can include inductive interpretation of the material or deductive approaches including systematic observation based on predefined coding categories. The collected observational data can subsequently be analysed using both qualitative and quantitative methods.

We will present and discuss the person-centred principles guiding a particular research project, the 'COMHOME' home care research project, particularly focusing on:

- how systematic observation using predefined categories for coding can represent the person perspective.
- methodological options and challenges linked to the interpretation of communication audio and video captured encounters.

Because all communication research embeds subjective interpretation, being a reflective practitioner as well as an objective researcher requires the ability both to reflect on one's activity and keep an analytic distance. This challenges the integration of empathic accuracy, compassion and cognitive clarity in person-centred communication research.

OVERVIEW OF THE COMHOME STUDY IN HOME HEALTHCARE

To preserve person-centred practices in home healthcare, insight into the communication practices in home healthcare is needed (Sundler *et al.*, 2016). Specific attention should be given to the challenges the nursing staff, in particular nursing assistants, face (Sundler *et al.*, 2016), how and which concerns service users express and how the nursing staff respond to these concerns. Nurse assistants and registered nurses provide healthcare for home-dwelling older people and the COMHOME project aims to provide knowledge on communication practices in home care (Hafskjold *et al.*, 2015). To address this purpose, service user–nurse and service user–nursing assistant communication during home care visits have been audio-recorded and explored using qualitative and quantitative methods of analysis. Moreover, a pilot-intervention to enhance nurses' emotional interactions with older persons using individual feedback was developed and tested (Veenvliet *et al.*, 2016). Based on the COMHOME study, a research-based online educational programme focusing on person-centred communication with older people (age ≥65), is being developed. The COMHOME study includes three European countries (Norway, Sweden and the Netherlands) and at a later point, the research project will be elaborated on to include practices from different countries.

PRINCIPLES OF PERSON-CENTREDNESS GUIDING THE STUDY

The definition of person-centredness by McCormack, Dewing and McCance (2011) is our point of departure for developing perspectives on person-centred communication: 'We define person-centred care as an approach to practice that is established through the formation and fostering of therapeutic relationships (...) [It] is underpinned by values of respect for persons, individual right to self-determination, mutual respect and understanding'. Recently, the term 'therapeutic relationships' has been changed to 'healthful relationships' (McCormack and McCance, 2016),which is a relationship that contributes to the promotion of health. The Aristotelian concept of eudaimonia or 'human flourishing', the highest human good, is also a key concept related to person-centred care in this theory. The Institute of Medicine suggests the following basis for person-centred care (IOM, 2001):

- Being respectful of patients' values, preferences, and expressed needs.
- Being coordinated and integrated.
- Providing information, communication and education.
- Ensuring physical comfort.
- Providing emotional support and relieving fear and anxiety.
- Involving family and friends.

Entwistle and Watt (2013) take this viewpoint a step further by suggesting a capabilities approach as the core of person-centred care, using the idea that 'treating patients as persons involves recognizing and cultivating their personal capabilities' as a point of departure. The authors recognise and suggest that healthcare professionals' capabilities are focused in three areas:

1. Respect and compassion.
2. Responsiveness to subjective experiences, unique biographies, identities and life projects.
3. Support for capabilities of autonomy.

These three perspectives on person-centred care all involve many aspects of communication, with the last perspective implying a relational ontology, which is learning about relational behaviours. The described frameworks are used to explore aspects of person-centred communication with older people in their private homes, in relation to the home care setting. Most people who require home care are older, depend on nursing care and personal assistance in their daily life activities. Many of them also have substantial physical disabilities, may be approaching the end of life, and may experience a divide between themselves and their healthcare providers.

METHODOLOGICAL APPROACH – USING SYSTEMATIC OBSERVATION

Emotional communication is of special interest in this study and especially communication of concerns and worries. For healthcare providers, detecting and relating to troubling negative emotions such as anger, fear and sadness is difficult (Sheldon, Barrett and Ellington, 2006; Eide, Sibbern and Johannessen, 2011; Zimmermann et al., 2011). However, detecting and relating to a service user's concerns regarding an existing health condition or life situation is of great importance for that person's well-being and provides foci for intervention (Zimmermann, Del Piccolo and Finset, 2007). Researching aspects of emotional communication is challenging. In 2003, an international group of communication researchers started to develop a common coding system for identifying different aspects of emotional communication and its role in the communication process. The system is called the Verona Coding Definitions for Emotional Sequences (VR-CoDES) (Zimmermann *et al.*, 2011) and includes a descriptive response system (Del Piccolo *et al.*, 2011). The two parts of the VR-CoDES are VR-CoDES Cues and Concerns and VR-CoDES Provider responses. The COMHOME study uses the VR-CoDES system to capture when service users utter negative emotions and when the care providers respond to these utterances. The VR-CoDES are described in short in the following paragraphs.

VR-CoDES C-C (cues and concerns)

The VR-CoDES C-C coding system provides a detailed description of *concerns*, i.e. clear expressions of a negative emotion, and specifications of seven different *cues*, i.e. ways of hinting or cueing emotionally important topics (Zimmermann *et al.*, 2011). A *concern* is defined as 'a clear and unambiguous expression of an unpleasant current or recent emotion where the emotion is explicitly verbalised'. A *cue* is defined as 'a verbal or non-verbal hint that suggests an underlying unpleasant emotion and would need clarification from the health provider'. The VR-CoDES C-C coding system has been validated using stimulated recall with people living with chronic pain (fibromyalgia). It has been found to have a high degree of ecological validity with referral to the person's worries and high sensitivity and specificity, giving a real picture of their major health and other life concerns (Eide *et al.*, 2011). The definitions of the different categories of cues and concerns are shown in Table 16.1.

Table 16.1 VR-CoDES Cues and Concerns, with examples from home care visits.

Definitions	Patients' expressions
Concern: a clear and unambiguous expression of an unpleasant current or recent emotion where the emotion is explicitly verbalised.	'My legs hurt so much; I am even afraid of touching myself'
Cue A Words or phrases in which the patient uses vague or unspecified words to describe his/her emotions.	'It is still very bad' (the nurse assistant had asked about the trembling of the patient's hand)
Cue B: verbal hints to hidden concerns (emphasising, unusual words, unusual description of symptoms, profanities, exclamations, metaphors, ambiguous words, double negatives, expressions of uncertainties and hope).	'I do not understand how this happened' (the stoma bag had leaked)
Cue C: words or phrases, which emphasise (verbally or non-verbally) physiological or cognitive correlates (regarding sleep, appetite, physical energy, excitement or motor slowing down, sexual desire, concentration) of unpleasant emotional states.	'Then I do not know how I can sleep tonight'
Cue D: neutral expressions that mention issues of potential emotional importance, which stand out from the narrative, background and refer to stressful life events and conditions.	
Cue E: a patient elicited repetition of a previous neutral expression.	'I have such trouble with my teeth, I have been to the dentist twice, but it doesn't get better'
Cue F: non-verbal cue: clear expressions of negative or unpleasant emotions (crying), or hint to hidden emotions (sighing, silence after provider question, frowning, etc.).	
Cue G: a clear and unambiguous expression of an unpleasant emotion which is in the past (more than one month ago) or is referred to an unclear period of life.	'That was terrible' (is talking about her father drowning when she was a child)

VR-CoDES P (provider responses)

The VR-CoDES P coding system provides a detailed description of the healthcare providers' *responses* to service users' negative emotions (Del Piccolo *et al.*, 2011). As communication is sequential, there is also a need to explore how providers respond to these expressed worries. Showing empathy is regarded as a key skill in interpersonal relationships; but there is a need to know how providers respond to concerns and also to understand what is a good way to respond in relation to immediate, intermediate and long-term health outcomes. The VR-CoDES P coding system categorises healthcare providers' responses to service user cues and concerns according to two major conceptual dimensions of the coding system:

1. Whether or not the provider provides space for further disclosure of the cue or concern.
2. Whether or not the response explicitly refers to the expressed cue or concern.

In this manner, a classification system of four main classes of provider responses is obtained. Each class is further subdivided into specific communication behaviours with a total of 17 separate categories (see Table 16.2).

Table 16.3 gives an example of the transcript of the dialogue between a woman (aged 86 years) receiving help from a male nurse assistant (aged 52 years) supporting her to prepare for the night. The transcript shows how a cue can be presented in a care situation by the person and the response from the nurse assistant as identified by VR-CoDES. The duration of this encounter was 18 minutes.

VR-CODES AS A PROCESS AND OUTCOME MEASURE – SOME REFLECTIONS

Audio and video recordings give rich data material, which can be investigated from several angles. This is an advantage compared with participatory observation as a method. Participatory observation gives a momentary observation relying on the notes taken during and after the observation. Having audio and video recordings of a real life situation allows more than one researcher, as well as the persons taking part in the encounters, to reflect on the encounter, thereby establishing a high degree of intersubjectivity.

VR-CoDES have been used in many studies to investigate the communication process and factors influencing this process (Vatne *et al.*, 2010; Eide *et al.*, 2011; Kale *et al.*, 2011; Grimsbø, Ruland and Finset, 2012; Finset, Heyn and Ruland, 2013;). In the COMHOME study VR-CoDES are used as a process to explore:

1. The nature of cues and concerns.
2. What promotes expressions of cues and concerns.
3. How the providers are responding to cues and concerns.
4. How their response affects the encounter.

Moreover, VR-CoDES have been used as an outcome measure of an intervention study of reflective practice (Veenvliet *et al.*, 2016), using both the number of cues and concerns expressed and the way the nurses respond to cues and concerns as outcome measures of reflective training.

Table 16.2 Overview of VR-CoDES - Provider Response.

Space given to the patient's perspective	Implicit or explicit referral to the cues and concerns (CC)	Behaviour definitions
Provide space	Implicit	1. *Silence* is when the provider provides a clear space or pause (3 seconds or more), allowing space for the patient to say more. 2. *Back-channel* is any response that provides space for the patient to say more or encourages further disclosure, through using a minimal prompt, or word, but not a full statement. 3. *Active invitation* is any response which explicitly seeks further disclosure or new information from the patient *about the cue or concern*, without making explicit reference to the content or the emotion/affect mentioned in the CC. 4. *Implicit empathy* is any response which provides space for further disclosure through having an empathic function, without asking explicitly for further clarification or specifically mentioning the nature or the emotion of the CC.
	Explicit	5. In *Content acknowledgement* the health provider explicitly refers to the *factual content* or topic of the CC by allowing space for further disclosure *without specifically seeking it and without referring explicitly to the emotional element*. 6. In *Content exploration* the health provider engages in behaviour which refers to the *factual content* or topic of the CC. 7. In *Affective acknowledgement* the health provider explicitly refers to the emotional aspect of the CC in the response. 8. *Affective exploration* is any health provider behaviour which explicitly picks up or refers to the *affective or emotional aspect* of the CC. 9. An *Empathic response* is a health provider behaviour that empathises with the patient predicament. The provider legitimises or shares the patient's emotion, with or without reference to provider's own feelings.
Reduce space	Implicit	10. *Ignoring:* the CC appears to be completely ignored. No reference whatsoever is made to either the content or the emotion of the CC. 11. *Shutting down* is a response that actively shuts down/moves away from the CC expressed, without making specific reference to it. 12. *Non-explicit information – advice is coded* when the health provider informs, gives advice or offers reassurance without referring explicitly to the CC, in a generic and non-specific way, with the function of non-inviting further disclosure. 13. *Acknowledgement* is any response which provides space for the patient to say more about a CC by 'non-specifically' acknowledging what has been said.
	Explicit	14. When *Switching* the health provider uses one of a number of behaviours which have the function of changing the frame of reference of the CC. The content or emotion of the CC MUST be clearly referred to. 15. *Postponement* is when the health provider suggests explicitly that further exploration of the CC is delayed. 16. *Information – advice* refers to an explicit response to the CC, which gives information or advice, or offers reassurance. 17. *Active blocking* is a response that expresses an explicit refusal on the part of the health provider to talk further about the CC, accompanied by a devaluation or disconfirmation of the patient or a refusal of what was said.

Table 16.3 Example of sequence of cues and nursing assistant's responses and VR-CoDES coding categories.

The service user and nursing assistant (NA) have discussed how the person has a bowl full of glasses that other care providers have left behind after their visit. The NA has, while discussing this topic, got the equipment ready for helping the person with her sore legs.

Setting	Time stamp	Actor	Utterance	VR-CoDES
NA helps the person with moisturising her legs and putting on new bandages.	6:15	NA	*Is it too tight*	
	6:16	Patient	*No it's not, it's not too tight*	
	6:17	NA	*Good*	
	6:19	Patient	*I feel so sorry for you who have to keep on caring for these legs*	Patient elicited cue A (vague or unspecified words to describe emotions)
	6:25	NA	*You feel sorry for us, yes?* (expressed with humour in tone of voice)	Explicit providing space – affective acknowledgement
	6:26	Patient	*You, yes, yuck, it is a shitty job*	Health provider elicited cue B (profanities)
	6:28	NA	*No, this* [these legs] *is not so bad*	Explicit reducing space – information advice
	6:29	Patient	*Oh, yes* (both NA and patient laugh)	
Conversation continuous				

VR-CODES – CONTRIBUTION TO THEORY DEVELOPMENT AND METHODOLOGICAL DEVELOPMENT

The VR-CoDES definitions were developed through a combination of previous research into the role of emotions in interpersonal relations and in communication research. A theory of basic emotions (Ekman, 2004) underpinned the development of the VR-CoDES. Using the VR-CoDES method in future research can contribute to the development of theory about the communication process related to the communication of concerns; and how the healthcare providers could respond in order to contribute to healthful relationships and promote health. Few studies have explored communication in a primary healthcare setting (the person's own home). This is a special setting and the COMHOME study can contribute to theory about person-centred communication with home-dwelling older people. A conversation analytical approach has been used to qualitatively explore sequences with departure from an expression of a cue or concern identified by VR-CoDES (Mellblom *et al.*, 2014). Moreover, VR-CoDES have also been used in innovative statistical analyses exploring sequential patterns and how factors such as comorbidity and deprivation influences patient–physician communication (Zhou *et al.*, 2015a; Zhou *et al.*, 2015b).

KEY LEARNING

Service user–healthcare provider communication is a core element of person-centred care. Therefore, service user expressions of worries are important moments in the communication between them and the health provider and can be captured by the VR-CoDES system in a valid and reliable way. Engaging with emotional aspects introduced by the service user can increase person-centred interactions by strengthening their relationship with the healthcare provider, gaining insight into what is important for the person and increasing a sympathetic presence from the healthcare provider. Investigating service user concerns may provide knowledge on how communication facilitates or hinders person-centred care.

REFERENCES

Del Piccolo, L., de Haes, H., Heaven, C. et al. (2011) Development of the Verona coding definitions of emotional sequences to code health providers' responses (VR-CoDES-P) to patient cues and concerns. *Patient Education and Counseling*, **82**, 149.

Eide, H. and Eide, T. (2007) *Kommunikasjon i relasjoner : samhandling, konfliktløsning, etikk* (2. rev. og utv. utg. ed.). Gyldendal akademisk, Oslo.

Eide, H., Eide, T., Rustøen, T. and Finset, A. (2011a) Patient validation of cues and concerns identified according to Verona coding definitions of emotional sequences (VR-CoDES): a video- and interview-based approach. *Patient Education and Counseling*, **82**, 156–162.

Eide, H., Sibbern, T., Egeland, T. et al. (2011b) Fibromyalgia patients' communication of cues and concerns interaction analysis of pain clinic consultations. *The Clinical Journal of Pain*, **27**, 602–610.

Eide, H., Sibbern, T. and Johannessen, T. (2011c) Empathic accuracy of nurses' immediate responses to fibromyalgia patients' expressions of negative emotions: an evaluation using interaction analysis. *Journal of Advanced Nursing*, **67**, 1242–1253.

Ekman, P. (2004) Happy, sad, angry, disgusted: everyone, whether they are from the highlands of Papua New Guinea or urban California, displays the same emotions in the same way. *New Scientist*, **184**(2467), S4.

Entwistle, V. and Watt, I. (2013) A capabilities approach to person-centered care: response to open peer commentaries on 'treating patients as persons: a capabilities approach to support delivery of person-centered care'. *The American Journal of Bioethics*, **13**, 1–4.

Finset, A., Heyn, L. and Ruland, C. (2013) Patterns in clinicians' responses to patient emotion in cancer care. *Patient Education and Counseling*, **93**, 80–85.

Grimsbø, G.H., Ruland, C.M. and Finset, A. (2012) Cancer patients' expressions of emotional cues and concerns and oncology nurses' responses, in an online patient–nurse communication service. *Patient Education and Counseling*, **88**, 36–43.

Hafskjold, L., Eide, T., Holmström, I. K. et al. (2016) Older persons' worries expressed during home care visits: exploring the content of cues and concerns identified by the Verona coding definitions of emotional sequence. *Patient Education and Counseling*, **99**, 1955–1963.

Hafskjold, L., Sundler, A. J., Holmström, I. K. et al. (2015) A cross-sectional study on person-centred communication in the care of older people: the COMHOME study protocol. *BMJ Open*, **5**, e007864.

Institute of Medicine [IOM] (2001) *Crossing the Quality Chasm: A New Health System for the 21st Century*. National Academy Press, Washington.

Kale, E., Finset, A., Eikeland, H.-L. and Gulbrandsen, P. (2011) Emotional cues and concerns in hospital encounters with non-Western immigrants as compared with Norwegians: An exploratory study. *Patient Education and Counseling*, **84**, 325–331.

McCormack, B., Dewing, J. and McCance, T. (2011) Developing person-centred care: addressing contextual challenges through practice development. *Online Journal of Issues in Nursing*, **16**, Manuscript 3. http://nursingworld.org/MainMenuCategories/ANAMarketplace/ANAPeriodicals/OJIN/TableofContents/Vol-16-2011/No2-May-2011/Developing-Person-Centred-Care.aspx (accessed 1 February 2017).

McCormack, B. and McCance, T. (2016) *Person-Centred Practice in Nursing and Healthcare: Theory and Practice*. Wiley Blackwell, Oxford.

Mellblom, A.V., Finset, A., Korsvold, L. *et al.* (2014) Emotional concerns in follow-up consultations between paediatric oncologists and adolescent survivors: a video-based observational study. *Psychooncology*, **23**, 1365–1372.

Sheldon, L.K., Barrett, R. and Ellington, L. (2006) Difficult communication in nursing. *Journal of Nursing Scholarship*, **38**, 141–147.

Sundler, A.J., Eide, H., Dulmen, S. and Holmström, I.K. (2016) Communicative challenges in the home care of older persons–a qualitative exploration. *Journal of Advanced Nursing*, **72**, 2435–44.

Vatne, T.M., Finset, A., Ørnes, K. and Ruland, C.M. (2010) Application of the Verona coding definitions of emotional sequences (VR-CoDES) on a pediatric data set. *Patient Education and Counseling*, **80**, 399–404.

Veenvliet, C., Eide, H., de Lange, M. and van Dulmen, S. (2016) Towards enhanced emotional interactions with older persons. Findings from a nursing intervention in home health care. *International Journal of Person-centred Medicine*, **3**, 191–199.

Zhou, Y., Humphris, G., Ghazali, N. *et al.* (2015a) How head and neck consultants manage patients' emotional distress during cancer follow-up consultations: a multilevel study. *European Archives of Otorhinolaryngology*, **272**, 2473–2481.

Zhou, Y., Lundy, J.-M., Humphris, G. and Mercer, S.W. (2015b) Do multimorbidity and deprivation influence patients' emotional expressions and doctors' responses in primary care consultations? An exploratory study using multilevel analysis. *Patient Education and Counseling*, **98**, 1063–1070.

Zimmermann, C., Del Piccolo, L., Bensing, J. *et al.* (2011) Coding patient emotional cues and concerns in medical consultations: the Verona coding definitions of emotional sequences (VR-CoDES). *Patient Education and Counseling*, **82**, 141–148.

Zimmermann, C., Del Piccolo, L. and Finset, A. (2007) Cues and concerns by patients in medical consultations: a literature review. *Psychological Bulletin*, **133**, 438.

Editors' Commentary

The importance of communication in all aspects of life can never be over-emphasised. In healthcare practice, communication is an essential skill that all healthcare professionals are educated in, as it cannot be assumed that it comes 'naturally' to us, given the complexity of most healthcare situations and encounters. However, communication practices in healthcare practice come under significant scrutiny, particularly when things go 'wrong'. Data arising from the review of complaints in healthcare demonstrate that poor communication is often a common theme of complaints and an underpinning reason for negative healthcare experiences. Whilst communication education is a central part of healthcare professional curricula and considerable investment is made in continuing professional development in communication practice, the reality is that many healthcare professionals struggle to communicate effectively. This is particularly the case in 'emotionally-laden' situations, e.g. breaking bad news, end of life conversations. While there is a lot of qualitative evidence exploring the make-up of such conversations and the challenges experienced by healthcare professionals, service users and families, it can be difficult to extract from these studies the key issues to be addressed. Further, quantitative studies into communication practices tend to take place in lab-like conditions where the stresses and stimuli are different from those experienced in real practice situations. The research presented by Eide and colleagues in this chapter shows a promising approach to 'getting under and inside' healthcare communication. The model of applying codes to particular expressions and utterances enables detailed coding of conversations, from which interpersonal connections can be delineated, further developed and analysed. Effective person-centred practice depends to a large extent on the interpersonal expertise of practitioners. However, in actual fact, we know little about person-centred interpersonal engagement beyond what has been extrapolated from other sources such as humanistic caring literature, communication studies and social-psychology. But do these general principles translate into a person-centred context or are there other/additional qualities that are needed? This is an important question for person-centred practice and the authors of this chapter identify methodological approaches that can help to answer it. The combination of ethnography, conversation analysis and a structured coding framework can enable detailed and systematic analysis of conversation in a variety of settings and can help to develop a deeper understanding of person-centred communication.

17 Introducing Sex and Gender-Sensitive Person-Centred Research

Stina Öresland and Sylvia Määttä

Reflective questions

1. In what way can this chapter be helpful in your own research?
2. In what way can the statement about common-sense knowledge be seen as a kind of bias?
3. What is the meaning of sex and gender insensitive person-centred research?

Breaking with prejudices and reconstructing the object of research requires a different way of seeing, in the light of which common-sense knowledge is reconstructed as a form of bias. (Oakley, 2000)

INTRODUCTION

For many years, the tradition of associating women with their biology and considering the male body as the norm has vitiated healthcare research (Oakley, 2000; Hammarström, 2007). Typically, healthcare research has often focused on men and the results generalised, regardless of whether they were relevant for women (Moerman and van Mens-Verhulst, 2004). As a response to scientific criticism, the more traditional 'one size fits all' approach to research emerged and women were little by little included in health research studies.

Today, researchers increasingly are aware of the importance of considering both women and men in their research. Editorials in scientific journals encourage paying attention to these issues in research and many reviewers require this before a paper is accepted for publication. Attempts at reconciling these issues have been made, for example in the growing area of gender medicine (Wijma, Smirthwaite and Swahnberg, 2010). However, there is still a need for significantly more work to be undertaken to address these issues adequately.

Person-Centred Healthcare Research, First Edition. Edited by Brendan McCormack, Sandra van Dulmen, Hilde Eide, Kirsti Skovdahl and Tom Eide.
© 2017 John Wiley & Sons Ltd. Published 2017 by John Wiley & Sons Ltd.

CONCEPTUAL CLARITY

Scholars and researchers are sometimes unfamiliar with the increasing body of knowledge on how sex and gender bias may influence research as well as clinical practice (Nowatzki and Grant, 2011; Mazure and Jones, 2015). Generally, the term sex is used in the context of biological characteristics, such as reproductive organs, chromosomes, hormonal patterns as well as processes at molecular and cellular levels distinguishing female from male bodies (Miers, 2002; Krieger, 2003; Hammarström, 2007). Gender, on the other hand, is often used when referring to culturally and socially constructed similarities and differences between the sexes. Thus, through cultural and social processes we all, repeatedly and methodologically, are 'doing gender' (West and Zimmerman, 1987). That is, gender is an expression of something a person 'does' according to societal rules and values, rather than something a person is or has. Consequently, gender is something that is never completed but is always in construction through social interaction. Doing gender means constructing differences between boys and girls, men and women, dissimilarities that are not biological, natural or essential. In addition, the terms *feminine* and *masculine* sometimes are assigned (Reese, 1995).

Some researchers have criticised the tendency to differentiate between gender and sex, fearing that attention to one might lead to unawareness of the other. They also fear that they will be ranked hierarchically in research (Hammarström, 2007). To avoid this, the interaction between sex and gender should always be considered in tandem since both contribute to influencing health and health outcomes (Nieuwenhoven and Klinge, 2010). According to Krieger (2003):

> *Not only can gender relations influence expression – and interpretation – of biological traits, but also sex-linked biological characteristics can, in some cases, contribute to or amplify gender differentials in health. (p. 653)*

The differentiation between sex and gender has also been problematised in queer theory. Judith Butler, one of the central exponents of queer theory, claimed that both sex and gender are constructed and depend on discursive practice (Butler, 2006). This includes sex that can be seen as an expression of essentialism, that is, sex understood as something internal and inherent. Queer theory, in part according to Zita (2000), is a reaction to considering that each sex comes with its own indispensable characteristics. In queer theory, the categorisation of gender and sexuality is contested. Advocates claim that identities are not fixed; identities consist of many components, and therefore cannot be labelled and categorised according to one characteristic. Central to queer theory is therefore a critique of heterosexuality and heteronormativity.

Recently, there has been increased awareness of the essential need to consider human life conditions, for example sex and gender, class, ethnicity and sexuality, in healthcare research (Anderson, 2000; Mill *et al.*, 2009; Van Herk, Smith and Andrew, 2011). In such an intersectionality paradigm it is assumed that no person is neutral – a sexless/genderless, classless and raceless person (for example), abstracted from the situated, social relations in which actual agents are embedded. According to intersectionality, life conditions constitute axes of power that are interrelated and cannot be seen as additive. Each of these axes of power construct and are constructed by the other (Glenn, 1999).

SEX AND GENDER PERSPECTIVES AND PERSON-CENTRED RESEARCH

With this background in focus, central to person-centred research is the stance that there is no entity, no 'person' without her/his life characteristics such as sex and gender. This awareness seems particularly important to person-centred research, as well as to person-centred care. To consider the uniqueness of the individual, understanding the life condition of the individual embedded in a social context, is at the heart of person-centred research. Thus, to neglect sex and gender in such an approach would be futile. Person-centred research must acknowledge that persons are socially and historically embedded, situated, contextual and relational, shaped by life conditions such as gender, ethnicity and race.

The aim of this chapter is therefore to combine sex and gender-sensitive research and person-centred research. We will introduce a sex and gender-sensitive person-centred research (SGPR) example, and elucidate some of the pitfalls of sex and gender-insensitive research.

TOWARDS SEX AND GENDER-SENSITIVE PERSON-CENTRED RESEARCH

Producing rigorous and valid person-centred research that incorporates sex and gender will lead to better science. To incorporate these aspects is critical, as sex and gender-insensitive person-centred research can lead to a number of biases that may distort the study and in the end jeopardise patient safety and quality of care. To enhance SGPR is important as 'old habits die hard, sex and gender-insensitive ways of doing research is passed on to a new generation of scientists. To be able to avoid sex and gender bias, researchers will have to act' (Neuwenhoven and Klinge, 2010, p. 316). Doing SGPR means to reflect on and make decisions on interweaving sex and gender in all steps and stages of a research process, and to realise that they often operate in tandem. In order to do this, the researcher must make a number of considerations when designing and conducting a study.

Doing a sex and gender-sensitive literature search

The SGPR process begins with the researcher's awareness of the distinction between sex and gender. The search strategy provides clues for relevant information for a sex and gender specific design. Such an approach can bring new and innovative results, expressed by Neuwenhoven and Klinge (2010): 'If our research addresses or identifies new, undocumented sex or gender differences it is innovative' (p. 318).

When planning a sex and gender-sensitive literature search strategy, the researcher must be aware of selection bias and consider:

- Which medical subject headings (MeSH) terms, heading terms and entry terms are appropriate to use, for example sex/gender, female/male, and femininity/masculinity – and how are these terms combined with the given area under study?

- Which databases are appropriate to use? Consider using for example Gender Equality Data and Statistics, Gender Studies Database.
- If inaccuracies or omissions exist in the literature, make note of these to avoid perpetuating this confusion.

Developing a sex and gender-sensitive study design

Following the SGPR process, the researcher ought to reflect on research question(s) and how these show the relevance of sex and gender. It is important to consider if the separate research question reflects similarities or differences between the sexes. In addition, gender effects might be of great importance and preclude relevant discussions, conclusions and recommendations for new practice.

Consider for example:

- Are the research questions able to explore similarities or differences between men and women?
- Have men and women different needs and expectations related to research outcomes?
- Is the research question or the hypothesis free from assumptions related to gender stereotypes?

Choosing sex and gender-sensitive research methods and data collection

Neither research methods nor methods of data collection are sex and gender-neutral. To avoid selection bias, a thoughtful reflection on the research population is essential. When describing the research population, gender and sex-neutral terms such as person, patients, individual, subjects and informants, etc. should be avoided, since there is a risk that such terms are more or less impregnated with values that might prejudice women or men. For example:

> In a review of two well-known international journals on pain research over the period of 2009–2012, a total of 1020 original abstracts were published. Sex and gender was used only in 246 abstracts. Some of these concerned studies on conditions affecting both men and women, for example fibromyalgia and low back pain. However, these studies included women only. On the other hand, studies on experimental pain included only men. (unpublished report)

To eschew selection bias, a description should specify the composition of men and women and how many men or women participated in the study. Differences between the sexes ought to be explored through a sex-disaggregated analysis. It is important to be aware of possible differences within and between men and women in a particular area, but also the causes and impacts of these differences. While there are many ways that sex can be included, gender is more difficult to reduce to variables that can be used in a statistical analysis, but its explanatory power can be massive.

Studies can also be flawed by performance bias, that is, the expectations of the researcher and the relationship between the researcher and the informants. Reflect on the following questions:

- Are both men and women included in the area of study? If not, consider inclusion and exclusion criteria.
- Are the variables and instruments appropriate for both men and women? If not, consider this limitation and consider modifying the variables and instruments if possible.
- How does the sex of the researcher and the sexes of the informants/subjects intersect?

Doing sex and gender-sensitive data analysis and reporting

To avoid detection bias, the SGPR analysis must address both sex and gender similarities and differences in text, and illustrate tables or figures suitable for both sexes. As in all research, reporting bias might be a challenge also in SGPR. When writing the results, there is a risk of for example underreporting, overgeneralisation or double standards. Overgeneralisation arises when a finding is generalised to groups other than the one studied. For example, it is not unusual that findings concerning men are generalised also for women. For example,

> in 1989, a trial focusing on low-dose aspirin for cardiovascular disease prevention was launched in the USA. The study enrolled 22 071 men and no women. Hence, the study left care providers uninformed on how low-dose medication would affect women and whether it would be preventive, have no effect or if it would harm women. (Mazure and Jones, 2015)

Overgeneralisation might also occur when using generic terms such as patient, subjects, humans, person, families, informants, etc. without clarifying which sex(es) are engaged. Overgeneralisation can also be present when using he, male, she, female, etc. when both sexes are intended. To avoid overgeneralisation, a non-sexist language is recommended. There is, for example, no 'single parent' without her/his sex; there is a woman or a man who is a 'single parent'.

Underreporting is, for example, present when sex and gender are not stated in the title or the abstract even if the text and tables show the sex of the included participants. In such cases, data from both sexes are collected, but sex similarities and differences are overlooked in the analysis. Underreporting is also at hand when sex or gender is not mentioned at all. For example, in a review of emergency medicine, Mazure and Jones (2015) found that: 'although 79% of the published studies from January 2006 to April 2009 reported gender as a demographic variable, only 18% examined health outcomes by gender' (p. 2).

There is a risk of using double standards when for example the same behaviour, characteristics, or attitudes are labelled differently when reporting the study on the basis of the person's sex. For example, the use of man and wife 'designates the man by sex and the woman by her marital status' (Neuwenhoven and Klinge, 2010, p. 319). Double standards might also be present when describing men and women as each other's opposite, for example men as active and women as passive; see for example 'sexual double standard is the notion that women in Western cultures are derogated men praised for engaging in identical sexual behaviours' (Zaikman and Marks, 2014, p. 333). Double standards can also be present when men's symptoms are taken as the norm. For example, describing symptoms as atypical when discussing symptoms of women's heart disease; such as in a study by Welch et al. (2012) where 'physicians view male sex as a "risk factor" but at times interpret women's symptoms as "atypical"' (p. 319).

Reflect on the following questions:

- When generalising results, are they based on research on both men and women or are they improperly used as a generic 'human person' model?
- What power relations can be observed while conducting the research? Between the researcher and the participants? Among the participants themselves?
- Are all images and illustrations sex and gender-balanced?
- Which strategies will reach both men and women?

A SEX AND GENDER-SENSITIVE CONCLUSION

In conclusion, an SGPR approach requires careful consideration of all stages of the research process. We have discussed underpinning principles at all stages of the research process. However, it is also important to consider how recommendations and implications from SGPR research are implemented in practice, as these same principles need to be applied in these activities and sex similarities/differences and gender effects should be considered. Similarly, when thinking about the education of health professionals, these principles and considerations should be included. Finally, much more work is needed in this field of research.

KEY LEARNING

There is a risk of person-centred research becoming sex and gender-insensitive. To prevent such a development, sex and gender-sensitive research has to be integrated with person-centred research. This might be a challenge and may not be so easy. However, an ethical approach that considers that persons are not neutral but live with their life conditions and circumstances is critical. By the study of a person's life conditions, person-centred research may gain new knowledge. This knowledge might in the long run lead to changes in clinical practice. In order to address and work with this awareness, a model for conducting sex and gender-sensitive research has been presented. Metaphorically, the request in this study is 'to see or not to see'. To be able to see what is not usually seen today in person-centred research, further research is necessary in the field of sex and gender-sensitive person-centred research within the healthcare system. A broad perspective on the subject is important.

REFERENCES

Anderson, J.M. (2000) Gender, 'race', poverty, health and discourses of health reform in the context of globalization: a postcolonial feminist perspective in policy research. *Nursing Inquiry*, **7**, 220–229.

Annandale, E. and Hammarström, A. (2011) Constructing the 'gender-specific body': A critical discourse analysis of publications in the field of gender-specific medicine. *Health*, **15**, 571–587.

Butler, J.P. (2006) *Gender Trouble – Feminism and the Subversion of Identity*. Taylor & Francis, New York.

Glenn, E.N. (1999) The social construction and institutionalization of gender and race: an integrative framework, in *Revisioning Gender* (eds M.M. Ferree, J. Lorber and B. Hess). Sage, London. pp. 3–43.

Hammarström, A. (2007) A tool for developing gender research in medicine: examples from the medical literature and work life. *Gender Medicine*, **24**, 123–132.

Krieger, N. (2003) Gender, sexes and health: what are the connections – and why does it matter? *International Journal of Epidemiology*, **32**, 652–657.

Mazure, C.M. and Jones, D.P. (2015) Twenty years and still counting: including women as participants and studying sex and gender in biomedical research. *BMC Women's Health*, **15**, 94.

Miers, M. (2002) Developing and understanding of gender sensitive care: exploring concepts and knowledge. *Journal of Advanced Nursing*, **40**, 69–77.

Mill, J.N., Jackson, E.R., Austin, W. *et al.* (2009) Accessing health services while living with HIV: intersections of stigma. *Canadian Journal of Nursing Research*, **41**, 168–85.

Moerman, C.J. and van Mens-Verhulst, J. (2004) Gender-sensitive epidemiological research: suggestions for a gender-sensitive approach towards problem definition, data collection and analysis in epidemiological research. *Psychology, Health and Medicine*, **9**, 41–52.

Nieuwenhoven, L. and Klinge, I. (2010) Scientific excellence in applying sex- and gender-sensitive methods in biomedical and health research. *Journal of Women's Health*, **19**, 313–321.

Nowatzki, N. and Grant, K. (2011) Sex is not enough: the need for gender-based analysis in health research. *Health Care for Women International*, **32**: 263–277.

Oakley, A. (2000) *Experiments in Knowing. Gender and Method in the Social Sciences.* Polity Press, Cambridge.

Reese, M. (1995) Leadership, gender, and emotionality: yesterday, today and tomorrow, in *Women as School Executives: Voices and Visions* (eds B. Irby and G. Brown). Texas Council of Women School Executives, Austin. pp. 94–98.

Van Herk, K.A., Smith, D. and Andrew, C. (2011) Examining our privileges and oppressions: incorporating an intersectionality paradigm into nursing. *Nursing Inquiry*, **18**, 29–39.

Welch, L.C., Lutfey, K.E., Gerstenberger, E. and Grace, M. (2012) Gendered uncertainty and variation in physicians' decisions for coronary heart disease: the double-edged sword of 'atypical symptoms'. *Journal of Health and Social Behavior*, **53**, 313–328.

West, C. and Zimmerman, D.H. (1987) Doing gender. *Gender and Society*, **1**, 125–151.

Wijma, B., Smirthwaite, G. and Swahnberg, K. (2010) *Genus och kön inom medicin och vårdutbildningar.* Studentlitteratur, Lund.

Zaikman, Y. and Marks, M.J. (2014) Ambivalent sexism and the sexual double standard. *Sex Roles*, **71**, 333–344.

Zita, J. (2000) Sexuality, in *A Companion to Feminist Philosophy* (eds A.M. Jaggar and I.M. Young). Blackwell Publishing, Oxford. pp. 307–320.

Editors' Commentary

The word 'person' is a loaded term with multiple meanings. In the world of person-centred practice it is used as a neutral term, avoiding association with other (more loaded) terms, such as patient and client. However, this chapter by Öresland and Määttä creates a pause for thought with regard to this terminology and raises our consciousness about the inherent dangers in so-called neutral terms. The authors make a strong case for sex and gender to be given an overt position in person-centred research and to ensure that sex and gender differences are understood and attended to at all stages of the research process. When planning this book, we were clear that a sex and gender perspective was needed, but the extent to which this was 'critical' to a comprehensive coverage of the subject area was less obvious! There is no doubt that sex and gender studies, queer theory and feminist epistemology have much greater prominence in research today, but are still treated like a 'minority' in the macro world of research. Yet there is little doubt that sex and gender differences play a huge part in the conduct of research, the dissemination of findings and the translation of findings into meaningful action. At the time of writing this commentary, we have witnessed the shocking shootings in the Orlando nightclub where 49 people were murdered (cf. https://en.wikipedia.org/wiki/2016_Orlando_nightclub_shooting). The reporting of this horrible event was overtly influenced by sex and gender thinking and the fact that it was a 'gay nightclub' dominated the public discourse in the media – even though not all the victims were gay! The effect of this discourse was one of isolating the significance of the shootings to a particular sub-set of the population (people who identify as LGBTQ+) and thus minimising the impact on the population as a whole. For some commentators, this was a positive effect as it highlighted that homophobia is 'alive and well' whilst for others it represented a negative stereotyping and a denigration of responsibility for the safety of all persons by the state irrespective of sexual orientation. This event raises many research questions that have a public health orientation and as Öresland and Määttä have suggested, applying the SGPR principles and processes presented by them could lead to interesting perspectives that may not be unearthed by other dominant approaches. The SGPR principles and processes hold great potential for paying attention to sex and gender in research studies, as they are not methodologically specific and can be applied in a variety of ways and in different contexts. This is an exciting opportunity for the field of person-centred research and one we should pay attention to. It is time for sex and gender to 'come out of the closet' of person-centred research!

18 Future Directions for Person-Centred Healthcare Research

Sandra van Dulmen, Brendan McCormack, Tom Eide, Kirsti Skovdahl and Hilde Eide

INTRODUCTION

This book offers a variety of chapters that all have one message in common; to do valuable healthcare research in the twenty-first century means to do research in a person-centred way. Person-centredness has evolved from a fuzzy concept with humanistic roots into a theoretical perspective that has conceptual clarity, operational principles and approaches to measurement, all of which means it can no longer be ignored when conducting healthcare research for, about and most importantly, with service users[1] in an ethical, reflective and methodologically robust way. As all of the chapters in this book have highlighted in a variety of ways, to get there, we need to relate to service users as persons and increase opportunities for them to feel empowered as citizens engaged in research and as active consumers of research outputs. The meaningful participation of service users in research is becoming much more established and significant progress has been made in moving beyond the tokenistic 'service user representative' on project advisory groups. Indeed, many research funders require the meaningful and active participation of service users as partners in research who are facilitated to be equal partners alongside professional researchers/academics. Further, the evolution of research governance frameworks in healthcare systems means that the assessment of project feasibility no longer stops at ensuring that recruitment strategies are ethical and that the study population is available. Contemporary approaches to the management of research consider the whole system including the potential burden of the research on staff in organisations, the ethical engagement with staff, consideration of 'payback' for staff participation and the need for proactive creative approaches to dissemination of findings. So, just like the way that person-centredness has evolved into a focus on the cultures of organisations and care settings, ensuring that person-centred principles are applied to all stakeholders, a similar evolution is happening in research. The diversity of the chapters in this book reflects this progress and provides a lens through which we can determine key principles and processes for progressing person-centred research. This final chapter attempts to synthesise the

---

[1] In this chapter the term 'service user' will be used to capture the variety of terms used when referring to service users, clients and patients.

Person-Centred Healthcare Research, First Edition. Edited by Brendan McCormack, Sandra van Dulmen, Hilde Eide, Kirsti Skovdahl and Tom Eide.

key messages and issues raised by the other chapters of the book regarding person-centred healthcare research and in doing this, addresses three questions:

1. Where were we?
2. Where are we now?
3. Where are we going from here?

WHERE WERE WE?

For a long time, research that focused on improving service users' quality of life or health outcomes was conducted without their involvement. Researchers set the agenda, decided on the outcomes of interventions to be pursued and reported their results for fellow-researchers or professionals without considering the point of view or added value for participants. Research was conducted in a science- or researcher-centred way. Through meta-analyses, findings were synthesised in a systematic way without considering the context in which the studies took place. The results of these endeavours were treated as evidence on which decisions were made for the most effective, but for service users, not automatically the most valued interventions. As Miles and Asbridge (2013) contend, this situation represents a perspective where the person is a part of the disease rather than seeing the disease as a part of the person. They suggest that this happens in healthcare research because of an obsession with classifying diseases and determining biological rationale for illnesses that may (and often do) have broader biopsychosocial origins.

In a similar way, randomised controlled trials were (and still are) the generally accepted route towards evidence-based medicine. Randomised controlled trials make an assumption of clinical equipoise; the treatments under study are perceived as equally desirable. However, for preference-sensitive treatments, like most treatments are, randomisation to a non-preferred treatment intervention complicates causal inferences and might even reduce external validity. This is even more so because characteristics of service users who have preferences may differ from those of service users who consent to randomisation, e.g. in terms of education (Feine, Awad and Lund, 1998). To pursue person-centred and values-based healthcare, changes in research methodology and related paradigm shifts were thus very much needed.

WHERE ARE WE NOW?

Creating connections

The plea in Western societies to cherish, respect and elicit the individual preferences and values of a person in need of help and to make a serious attempt to consider how an individual health professional can support a person in this process has really moved healthcare forward. We see these changes reflected in the different ways that are advocated when doing research in this context. In Chapter 4, for example, the influence of the person of the researcher is considered which indicates that doing research in a person-centred way has relevance that goes far beyond the person of the service user. The authors identify a key principle of person-centred research being 'connectivity', which focuses on co-action of researchers and participants. Operating such a principle requires a radical shift away from the traditional stance of the 'evidence speaking for itself' and thus to be applied irrespective of stated preferences. Instead, connectivity, as the authors argue, demands the making explicit of underlying values and goals and engagement with relational processes. In previous research, McCormack (2003) identified five conditions for doing person-centred research, the first of which is '*Informed Flexibility*', defined as: *the facilitation of decision-making through information sharing and the integration of new information into established perspectives.*

This condition is similar to that of connectivity. It highlights the need for researchers to be active facilitators of engaged relationships with research participations. Working with values and being authentic in their operationalisation demands for new information related to the project to be integrated into prior information so that participants can actively engage in decisions and reconsider their personal goals of participation. McCormack (2003) suggested that it requires the researcher to have a flexible approach to the way participation is negotiated and to be able to use a variety of conversational approaches in doing this. Being person-centred requires the researcher to be sensitive to the practice setting and the variety of unpredictable challenges that might arise. However, as the authors of Chapter 4 remind us – 'there is no recipe for doing person-centred research and no easy way out of relational obstructions…'. However, strategies that might enable this to happen include: (i) having a repertoire of conversational approaches in negotiating the research processes, and (ii) being flexible in the organisation of the research and adopting a non-routine approach to the conduct of the research.

In Chapter 5 creating connections is further elaborated upon when applying technology, for which it is important to consider and secure different aspects of person-centredness and regularly monitor end users' needs, experiences and perspectives. The use of PROMS (Patient Reported Outcome Measures) and PREMS (Patient Reported Experience Measures) is increasingly considered as standard research methodology. It is not in the gift of a researcher or even a health professional to decide what the most valuable outcome of an intervention is, but it is up to service users to decide. In this process, the researcher's role is to set and guard the methodological boundaries and playground. Besides, service users are increasingly involved in research projects as members of a project group and have, as such, a say in the way their fellow-service users are involved and approached. Through service user organisations, they furthermore set research agendas and act as reviewers of project grants. In this way, service user involvement, the burden of participating in research projects and the relevance of a research project from a service user point of view are being safeguarded and, as a positive side-effect, researchers learn how to explain and promote their research projects to lay persons. Paying attention to the active engagement of service users in research brings to life a second condition of person-centred research – '*Mutuality*', defined as: *the recognition of the others' values as being of equal importance in decision-making.*

The research literature places heavy emphasis on the values of the researcher and depending on the research design, the explication of values is seen as either an appropriate or inappropriate activity. In person-centred research, values are central, are explicit, are considered and are acted upon, and this condition makes explicit the need for considering the values held by all participants in research decision-making. Knowing the underpinning values held by service users, nurses, clinical teams and other participants is essential to effective person-centred decision-making. McCormack (2003) suggests that researchers need to make time to get to know (as far as possible) the values held by potential participants and shared by clinical teams. Strategies that might enable this to happen include: (i) a willingness to listen to and understand participants' expression of their values and to hold these central to decision-making; (ii) a willingness to work with the perceptions and understandings of others and to consider these perceptions in the overall research plan; and (iii) a willingness to learn from the relationships established with participants. Listening to and respecting service users is one of the key components of person-centred care (Mezzich *et al.*, 2013).

Considering context

Over the past 10 years or so, the importance of 'context' on the processes and outcomes of research has been increasingly recognised. Even the most purist trialist increasingly recognises that the outcomes of healthcare research are embedded in contexts. Advances in process evaluation that recognise the complexity of healthcare contexts and the need for sophisticated data collection methods that 'dig deep' into enablers and hinderers of trial effectiveness demonstrate greater commitment to understanding context among researchers. Greenhalgh *et al.* (2016) in a letter to the *British Medical Journal (BMJ)* make a convincing plea for academic journals to be respectful of qualitative research approaches that are central to digging deep in context. Greenhalgh *et al.* were responding to an 'article rejection' letter in the *BMJ* which stated that the paper was rejected because it was qualitative in nature and qualitative research was of low priority. The authors of the letter cited numerous examples where qualitative research added richness to studies, provided explanations of effectiveness or lack of effectiveness of interventions and demonstrated the impact of individuals, teams and contexts on research outcomes. In this book, the importance of methodologies that illuminate and illustrate contextual influences, explain rationale underpinning decisions, describe contextual factors and demonstrate psychosocial causations are demonstrated. Examples of this include: using ethnography to understand the mental health needs of older people (Chapter 12), observational studies to better understand person-centred communication (Chapter 16), narrative methodologies to connect with hard to reach groups (Chapter 10) and participatory research as a way of engaging with people living with dementia (Chapter 7). Other methodologies including realistic reviews (cf. Rycroft-Malone *et al.*, 2014), the 'N of 1' trial (Schork, 2015) and step-wedged designs (Hemming *et al.*, 2015) are other ways of considering the influence of the context in which a service user or healthcare as a whole operates when interpreting research findings.

Paying attention to context in these ways illustrates McCormack's (2003) condition of 'Transparency' for person-centred research, defined as: *the making explicit of intentions and motivations for action and the boundaries within which decisions are set.*

The condition of transparency requires researchers to engage with research participants in decision-making processes and to gain an understanding of the issues that might directly impact on potential participants and to interpret the outcomes of research in ways that do justice to understanding research participants' life-worlds. This potentially yields more ecologically valid conclusions. For example, to account for service users' treatment preferences, 'patient preference trials' have been proposed (Quang *et al.*, 2014). Differences in service user characteristics (e.g. more female and allochthonous persons with a depression, more older and autochthonous persons with chronic pulmonary airways disease) make it possible to study service user characteristics in relationship with treatment preferences and outcomes (van der Wurff *et al.*, 2004; Uijen *et al.*, 2008). Because preferences may interact with random assignment to influence outcome (Bower *et al.*, 2005; Cuijpers *et al.*, 2015), it is especially relevant to consider preferences in treatments that cannot be blinded (Preference Collaboration Review Group, 2008), like counselling and lifestyle interventions.

Strategies that researchers can use to operationalise the condition of transparency include: (i) being clear about professional boundaries in decision-making; (ii) understanding different ways in which researcher responsibility and accountability need to be operationalised; (iii) adopting a person-centred approach to risk assessment and risk taking when planning for service-user participation in research; and (iv) being willing to make explicit intent and motivation for actions.

The 'person' in the data

These examples of alternative research designs and methodology make clear that important steps have been taken to turn the highly protocolised research standards into meaningful person-centred approaches. The necessary paradigm shift has not been fully accomplished yet – and the extent to which it can ever be fully realised is questionable given the paradigm wars that continue to rage! In 2015, the World Health Organization (2007) launched their new strategy for securing people-centred and integrated health services which challenges future person-centred and people-centred healthcare services and associated research especially but not exclusively, in primary healthcare (Epperly *et al.*, 2015). In a recent editorial, Miles and Asbridge (2016) challenged some of the disease-orientated focus on health by the WHO in the context of the global growth in long-term conditions. They argue that a person-centred approach is needed to tackle long-term conditions:

> ... *when the indicated pharmacological and technical interventions have been instituted, it cannot realistically be concluded that this is all there is to do and that all of the other manifestations of the illness are somehow 'someone else's concern' and not that of the attending clinicians. (p. 2)*

This challenge to the dominant position of 'cure' and a call for a greater focus on a holistic and person-centred approach to population health and management of long-term conditions, not only poses challenges for health systems, but also for healthcare research in terms of research foci, methodological processes and intended outcomes of research activities.

Person-centred healthcare research needs to focus on the challenges that hinder these kind of practices and to monitor research methodologies, designs and projects that best serve the purpose of fostering person-centred healthcare across the lifespan. This is not to suggest that research that rightly focuses on finding cures for some of the most prominent public health challenges globally should not be a priority, as this is necessary. However, this focus alone is not sufficient in addressing global health challenges in ways that recognise the humanity of persons as well as the psychological, behavioural and social dimensions of health. The need to humanise healthcare is well recognised in both the work of the WHO and by public health academics (for an overview of definitions and activities see Harding, Wait and Scrutton, 2015). How individuals respond to and experience the impacts of disease and illness is a critical issue in managing long-term conditions (for example) but is also a complex area of research – because epidemiological data directs a particular course of health action doesn't mean that individual responses to these same diseases and illnesses can be globalised in the same way. This issue is consistent with McCormack's (2003) condition of '*Sympathetic Presence*' in research, defined as: *an engagement that recognises the uniqueness and value of the individual, by appropriately responding to cues that maximise the person's opportunity to participate/not participate.*

Working with sympathetic presence in research demands an integrative, collaborative and inclusive approach to research design. Sympathetic presence in this context focuses on balancing 'big data' with individual experience, preference, choice and decision-making. Thus researchers working in a person-centred way need to be sensitive to these different dimensions and to cues that participants may give regarding their preferred choices and decisions. However, as McCormack (2003) noted, 'given the power relationships at play, this may not be easy for participants to do'. Strategies that researchers can use to operationalise the condition of sympathetic presence include: (i) recognition of the power of language and the effects of language on the autonomy of the other person; (ii) the use of appropriate questioning styles that facilitate the setting of a person-centred conversation; (iii) considering ways in which studies can involve individual perspectives alongside generalisable data.

Paradigmatic synergies

There is little doubt that if researchers are going to consider person-centredness in their practice, then there is a need for methodological pluralism. While at the level of concept and theory it is likely that there will always be different perspectives on the importance or not of particular methodologies. This critical debate and discourse is to be welcomed as it creates spaces for shared learning and understanding – which from a person-centred perspective can enable new approaches to the integration of methodological principles and their operationalisation in practice, whilst recognising that the knowledge area that will dominate the particular research focus is dependent on the research question or questions that need to be solved and answered.

Paradigmatic synergies can be focused on a system level, a group level or an individual level and need to integrate knowledge from natural science, social science and the humanities. Natural sciences, social sciences and humanities are represented by quite different ontological and epistemological positions. Kagan (2009) has described the differences between the sciences on the following dimensions: (i) the primary questions asked; (ii) the sources of evidence the inferences are based on and the degree of control; (iii) primary vocabulary; (iv) the influence of historical conditions; (v) ethical influence; (vi) dependence on outside support; (vii) work conditions; (viii) contribution to national economy; and (ix) criteria for beauty. Kagan's conclusion is that the borders between the science areas have not been broken down and those differences continue to exist today to an even larger degree. However, professionals working in healthcare draw on all these science areas, but they are often linked more to one than another. Physicians draw heavily on empirical knowledge from the natural sciences, but also draw on social science when it comes to working with the service user, governed by the biopsychosocial model. Social workers are more inclined to draw on knowledge from social science and humanities. Psychologists, however, started out from philosophy and humanities and now build more and more knowledge on methodologies from the natural science paradigm, especially linked to the knowledge of neuropsychology. This psychological shift has changed perspectives on how the human body and especially the brain evolves and changes throughout life. Because of the unique position that nursing holds in healthcare provision, nursing knowledge is by necessity 'eclectic' drawing on natural sciences, social sciences and humanities. The integration of the areas in nursing practice, education and research enables nurses to focus on the health-related experiences of persons in context, the determining of appropriate interventions and practices and the adoption of holistic person-oriented engagements. Illustrating the different point of departure from different healthcare professional perspectives demonstrates the challenges we all face in holding the person central and designing research activities from the perspective of the person. Paradigmatic pluralism requires a shift of emphasis in the starting point of our research and in particular perhaps, a reorientation of the questions we ask and consider priority. From a person-centred perspective this reorientation is consistent with McCormack's (2003) condition of *'Negotiation'* in research, defined as: *participation through a research framework that values the views of the participant as a legitimate basis for decision-making.*

As Kagan (2009) reminds us, many of the paradigmatic differences arise from the primary question asked by researchers. This primary question then directs all subsequent decision-making regarding methodology and methods. However, in healthcare practice, few if any conditions, illnesses, diseases or experiences can be answered by a single question demanding a particular scientific perspective. Even if there exists a dominant question, there may be a variety of subquestions that lend themselves to complementary areas of inquiry. Further, if we are to argue that it is important to adopt a person-centred approach to our research, then determining research questions needs to be the starting point for that. Increasingly research funders require researchers to engage with service users in determining research questions. In the UK for example, an organisation called 'The James Lind Alliance' (JLA) operates to 'change the way research funding is granted, and to raise awareness of research questions which are of direct relevance and potential benefit to patients and the clinicians who treat them' (http://www.jla.nihr.ac.uk/about-the-james-lind-alliance/). Funded by the UK National Institute for Health Research (NIHR), the JLA believes that:

- addressing uncertainties about the effects of a treatment should become accepted as a routine part of clinical practice and
- patients, carers and clinicians should work together to agree which, among those uncertainties, matter most and deserve priority attention.

It has become routine practice to focus on JLA prioritised questions when applying for funding to organisations such as the NIHR. Ensuring that service users are playing a key role in informing what research is undertaken is a significant step forward. In addition, significant progress has been made in ensuring that service users are treated equally in the conduct of research. Organisations like 'Involve' (http://www.invo.org.uk/) have produced guidelines for paying service users as research participants and ensuring that they are treated as equal partners in research. Further, advances in peer-research, i.e. service users as researchers (https://www.publicengagement.ac.uk/do-it/techniquesapproaches/peer-led-qualitative-research) are rapidly developing. All of these strategic developments are changing the landscape of research and the engagement of service users in research decisions and processes. These strategic developments illustrate engagement in action and demonstrate the condition of negotiation being achieved. These strategies can be summarised into the following principles:

- Working within a collaborative framework that values the 'subjective' views of the person equally with other 'objective' perspectives.
- Establishing a negotiation framework in the planning and doing of the research that seeks to continuously clarify persons' values and priorities.
- Recognition of the interdependence of people in society and thus the need to consider different methodologies to understand the nature of that interdependence.

In this section we have highlighted some issues in the development of person-centred research and have identified examples of existing good practice in the field, many of which have been written about in this book. Clearly, there is still a long way to go to bridge paradigms and professional silos, as well as building a shared person-centred view of research.

WHERE ARE WE GOING FROM HERE?

This book is being produced at a time when there is an unprecedented interest in the development of person-centred research approaches. The collection of examples provided in this book that challenge existing paradigms and methods (see for example Chapters 3, 4, 5, 6 and 7) and propose new ways of engaging in the planning and conduct of research as well as the role of the researcher are important contributions to this development. Other chapters provide key insights into how researchers can engage in person-centred research or at least consider the place of 'the person' in research designs with a variety of foci including ICT (Chapter 13), workforce planning (Chapter 9), leadership development (Chapter 8), working with people living with dementia (Chapter 7), communication studies (Chapter 16), supporting learning (Chapter 14), vision (Chapter 15), gender studies (Chapter 17) and health promotion (Chapter 11) and in a variety of settings, including community care (Chapter 12), nursing homes (Chapter 10) and acute care (Chapter 8). All of these chapters provide a significant body of knowledge upon which to build a future agenda for the ongoing development of person-centred research in healthcare.

In Chapter 3, Angie Titchen, Shaun Cardiff and Stian Biong present what they refer to as a 'beginning epistemological and ontological framework for person-centred research'. In considering this framework in the context of the rest of the chapters in this book and the issues raised so far in this chapter, it is clear that many of the chapters relate with, connect to and illustrate the framework in action. Titchen, Cardiff and Biong suggest that the framework should have four constructs, derived from the person-centred framework of McCormack and McCance (2010):

1. *Person-centred research environment:* consideration of the contextual influences on the relationships researchers have with participants, their own being and the research process.
2. *Pre-requisites for person-centred research:* focuses especially on 'reflexivity'. A reflexive researcher should be able to articulate and reflect on their personal values, beliefs and needs (being and becoming) and from this act with a moral intention of doing 'good'.
3. *Person-centred research processes:* a number of processes characterise person-centred research, all of which contribute to the creation of (virtual) safe, critical and creative communicative spaces.
4. *Person-centred research outcomes:* participant and researcher wellbeing/flourishing during (and after) the research period.

Like the authors of Chapter 3, we would also conclude that there is much potential in further developing and testing this framework through international research collaborations and partnership working with research funders, advocacy organisations and healthcare practitioners.

CONCLUSION

Despite all that has been achieved so far, we are only at the very beginning of the development of person-centred healthcare research. The big challenge is to carry out this development while maintaining the rigour demanded of high quality research. These are not opposing agendas, as after all, conducting healthcare research in a person-centred way does not come easy but poses higher demands on research skills and resources. So, what's next? How can we achieve sustainable person-centred methodology in our healthcare research? There is no doubt that developing rigorous research methodologies will continue to be the raison d'etre of high quality research design in testing new interventions, evaluating effectiveness of interventions, determining the value of particular approaches to care and treatment, as well as informing healthcare developments. Starting from a person-centred perspective does not detract from those agendas, but instead demands researchers and research funders to consider the 'voice of the person' in all stages of the research as a complementary addition to established designs. Service users' voices can be used as a way of weighing the relevance and validity of rigorously obtained findings. In addition, more research is needed to examine the feasibility and efficacy of centring clinical trial designs (e.g. patient preference trials) around service users' preferences, i.e. around their expectations and values of the process and outcome of specific treatment interventions. Research into the experiences of service users is increasing and new methodological approaches are continually evolving that enable creative, holistic and ultimately person-centred approaches to evaluating experience to be realised. Research into the different contextual factors that impact on patient-outcome is also much more established in healthcare research as well as increasing research into the dynamic relationship between staff 'ways of being' and patient outcome/experience. However, there is no doubt that the biggest challenge facing the development of person-centred research is the paradigm shift that is needed to accomplish these developments. As a number of chapters in this book illustrate, some movement has been created but these need to be nurtured, supported and further developed in order to bring about a transformation of the nature of research in healthcare and the focus on person-centredness.

REFERENCES

Bower, P., King, M., Nazareth, I. *et al.* (2005) Service user preferences in randomized controlled trials: conceptual framework and implications for research. *Social Science and Medicine*, **61**, 685–695.

Cuijpers, P., Karyotaki, E., Andersson, G. *et al.* (2015) The effects of blinding on the outcomes of psychotherapy and pharmacotherapy for adult depression: a meta-analysis. *European Psychiatry*, **30**, 685–693.

Epperly, T., Roberts, R., Rawaf, S. *et al.* (2015) Person-centered primary health care: now more than ever. *The International Journal of Person Centered Medicine*, **5**, 53–59.

Feine, J.S., Awad, M.A. and Lund, J.P. (1998) The impact of service user preference on the design and interpretation of clinical trials. *Community Dentistry and Oral Epidemiology*, **26**, 70–74.

Greenhalgh, T., Annandale, E., Ashcroft, R. *et al.* (2016) An open letter to *The BMJ* editors on qualitative research. *British Medical Journal*, **352**, i563.

Harding, E., Wait, S. and Scrutton, J. (2015) The state of play in person-centred care: a pragmatic review of how person-centred care is defined, applied and measured, featuring selected key contributors and case studies across the field. The Health Policy Partnership, London. http://www.healthpolicypartnership. com/wp-content/uploads/State-of-play-in-person-centred-care-12-page-summary-Dec-2015-FINAL-PDF.pdf (accessed 1 February 2017).

Hemming, K., Haines, T.P., Chilton, P.J. *et al.* (2015) The stepped wedge cluster randomised trial: rationale, design, analysis, and reporting. *British Medical Journal*, **350**, h391.

Kagan, J. (2009) *The Three Cultures: Natural Sciences, Social Sciences, and The Humanities in the 21st Century*. Cambridge University Press, Cambridge.

McCormack, B. (2003) Researching nursing practice: does person-centredness matter? *Nursing Philosophy*, **4**, 179–188.

McCormack, B. and McCance, T. (2010) *Person-centred Nursing: Theory, Models and Methods*. Wiley Blackwell, Oxford.

Mezzich, J.E., Appleyard, J.E., Botbol, M. *et al.* (2013) Ethics in person centered medicine: conceptual place and ongoing developments. *The International Journal of Person-Centred Medicine*, **3**, 255–257.

Miles, A. and Asbridge, J.E. (2013) Contextualizing science in the aftermath of the evidence-based medicine era: on the need for person-centered health care. *European Journal for Person Centered Health care*, **1**, 285–289.

Miles, A. and Asbridge, J.E. (2016) The chronic illness problem. The person-centered solution. *European Journal for Person Centered Health Care*, **4**, 1–5.

Preference Collaborative Review Group (2008) Service users' preferences within randomised trials: systematic review and service user level meta-analysis. *BMJ*, **337**, a1864.

Quang, A. le, Doctor, J.N., Zoellner, L.A. and Feeny, N.C. (2014) Cost-effectiveness of prolonged exposure therapy versus pharmacotherapy and treatment choice in posttraumatic stress disorder (the optimizing PTSD treatment trial): a doubly randomized preference trial. *Journal of Clinical Psychiatry*, **75**, 222–230.

Rycroft-Malone, J., Burton, C., Hall, B. *et al.* (2014) Improving skills and care standards in the support workforce for older people: a realist review. *BMJ Open*, **4**, e005356.

Schork, N.J. (2015) Time for one-person trials. *Nature*, **520**, 609–611.

Uijen, A.A., Schermer, T.R.J., Hoogen, H.J.M. van den *et al.* (2008) Prevalentie en zorgconsumptie bij astma en COPD in relatie tot etniciteit. *[Prevalence of and health care consumption for asthma and COPD in relation to ethnicity]. Ned Tijdschr Geneeskd*, **152**, 1157–1163.

World Health Organization (2007) *People-centred Health Care: A Policy Framework*. Retrieved from: http://www.wpro.who.int/health_services/people_at_the_centre_of_care/documents/ENG-PCIPolicy Framework.pdf (accessed 1 February 2017).

Wurff, F.B. van der, Beekman, A.T., Dijkshoorn, H. *et al.* (2004) Prevalence and risk-factors for depression in elderly Turkish and Moroccan migrants in the Netherlands. *Journal of Affective Disorders*, **83**, 33–41.

Index

Page numbers in *italics* refer to figures.
Page numbers in **bold** refer to tables.

acknowledgement, in provider responses, **196**
action plan templates, *135*
action research, *see also* participatory action
    research
  emancipatory, 157
  ethnography in, 151
  evaluation systems, 111
  leadership, 101, 102–104, 106–110
  learning, 110
  narrative approach, 133, 134
action spirals, leadership research, 107
active blocking, in provider responses, **196**
active invitation, in provider responses, **196**
active learning (Dewing), 134
acute care unit, older people, 106–110
addiction *see* substance abuse
adverse events, RAFAELA® system on, 127
affective acknowledgement, in provider
    responses, **196**
affective exploration, in provider responses, **196**
agendas, system *vs* patient, 12
alarms (passive position alarms), 91, 160–161
alcohol, ENGAGE intervention, 77
alongside, leading from, 110
Alzheimer Society (Canada), 9
anxiety
  challenge causing, 169
  Johns on, 138
apathy, as defence, 80
Aristotle, 22, 23
aspirin (low-dose), women excluded, 205
atomistic fallacy, 185
attentiveness, 53, 107
audio recordings, 196
austerity (budget cuts), 119, 153
Australia, organisations, 7–8, 9
authenticity, 177
autonomy, 53

respect for, 5
technology on, 65–66
axes of power, 202

back-channel provider responses, **196**
balancing (of needs), 108
bandaging of legs, **197**
bedrocks *see* worldviews
Behavioural and Psychological Symptoms of
    Dementia, model, 87
behind, leading from, 110
being
  doing *vs*, 88
  narrative, 133, 136–137
  researchers, 55
being in the world (Heidegger), 138
'being there' (presencing), 38, 107
benchmarking and benchlearning, 120
benchmarking reports, 126–127
biographies, 5
blocking (active), in provider responses, **196**
blur (visual), 184
bottom-up method, PAONCIL method as, 121
brain infarcts, nursing intensity, 125
bravery, personal, 5
British Medical Journal, qualitative research
    and, 212
Buber, M., 24, 26, 88
budget cuts, 119, 153
business models, person-centredness *vs*, 7
Buurtzorg model, community nursing, 8

Canada
  Alzheimer Society, 9
  Ottawa Charter for Health Promotion, 141, 142
capabilities approach (Entwistle and Watt), 193
capacities of persons, 23, 89
cardiovascular disease, sex and gender, 205

Person-Centred Healthcare Research, First Edition. Edited by Brendan McCormack, Sandra van Dulmen,
Hilde Eide, Kirsti Skovdahl and Tom Eide.
© 2017 John Wiley & Sons Ltd. Published 2017 by John Wiley & Sons Ltd.